Birth Territory and Midwifery Guardianship

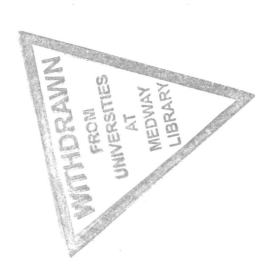

Commissioning Editor: Mairi McCubbin
Development Editor: Sheila Black
Project Manager: Krishnan Balakrishnan
Designer: George Ajayi

Birth Territory and Midwifery Guardianship

Theory for Practice, Education and Research

Edited by

Kathleen Fahy BN MEd PhD RM RN

Professor of Midwifery, University of Newcastle, Newcastle, NSW, Australia

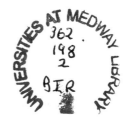

Maralyn Foureur BA GradDip Clin Epidem PhD RM RN

Professor of Midwifery, University of Technology, Sydney and Northern Sydney Central Coast Health, Sydney, NSW, Australia

Carolyn Hastie DipTeach GradDipPHC ILBC RM RN

Midwifery Manager, Belmont Birthing Service, Obstetrics and Gynaecology Department, John Hunter Hospital, Hunter New England Health, Newcastle, NSW, Australia

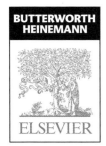

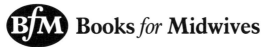

Books *for* Midwives

EDINBURGH LONDON NEW YORK OXFORD PHILADELPHIA ST LOUIS SYDNEY TORONTO 2008

**BUTTERWORTH
HEINEMANN**
ELSEVIER

Books for Midwives
An imprint of Elsevier Limited

First published 2008

ISBN 978-0-7506-8870-3

British Library Cataloguing in Publication Data
A catalogue record for this book is available from the British Library

Library of Congress Cataloging in Publication Data
A catalog record for this book is available from the Library of Congress

Notice
Neither the Publisher nor the Editors assume any responsibility for any loss or injury
and/or damage to persons or property arising out of or related to any use of the
material contained in this book. It is the responsibility of the treating practitioner,
relying on independent expertise and knowledge of the patient, to determine the best
treatment and method of application for the patient.

The Publisher

ELSEVIER your source for books,
journals and multimedia
in the health sciences
www.elsevierhealth.com

Working together to grow
libraries in developing countries
www.elsevier.com | www.bookaid.org | www.sabre.org

ELSEVIER   BOOK AID International   Sabre Foundation

The
publisher's
policy is to use
**paper manufactured
from sustainable forests**
II

Printed in China

Contents

Contributors

Pat Brodie DMid MN RN RM
Professor of Maternity Practice Development & Research, University of Technology, Sydney & Sydney Southwest Area Health Service, Broadway, NSW, Australia

Kathleen Fahy BN MEd PhD RM RN
Professor of Midwifery, University of Newcastle, Newcastle, NSW, Australia

Maralyn Foureur BA GradDip Clin Epidem PhD RM RN
Professor of Midwifery, University of Technology, Sydney and Northern Sydney Central Coast Health, Sydney, NSW, Australia

Carolyn Hastie DipTeach GradDipPHC ILBC RM RN
Midwifery Manager, Belmont Birthing Service, Obstetrics and Gynaecology Department, John Hunter Hospital, Hunter New England Health, Newcastle, NSW, Australia

Nicky Leap DMid MSc RM
Professor of Midwifery Practice Development and Research, University of Technology, Sydney, Broadway, NSW, Australia

Bianca Lepori MA
Architect, Rome, Italy

Michel Odent MD
Director, Primal Health Research Centre, London, UK

Lesley Page BA MSc PhD RM RN FRCM(Honorary)
Visiting Professor of Midwifery, Nightingale School of Nursing and Midwifery, King's College, London, UK

Jennifer A. Parrat BHLthSci MMid(US) RM FACM
Midwife and PhD Candidate, University of Newcastle, Newcastle, NSW, Australia

Preface

Folklore in all cultures has been clear about the necessity of protecting childbearing women in environments in which they feel safe and nurtured, but we have lost touch with this in the West. This book is about the impact that the environment has on the childbearing woman and her baby and, by extension, all families and all communities. It develops a new theoretical approach to understanding birth from a woman-centred midwifery perspective or paradigm. The obstetric paradigm that is commonly used to describe, explain and predict birthing posits that birthing can be understood and improved upon by the use of a reductionistic, disembodied and mechanistic theory. In the obstetric paradigm, the process of labour is described as involving three core concepts, referred to as the three Ps: the powers (uterine contractions) the passages (maternal pelvis and soft tissues) and the passenger (the fetus which is thought of as an inert package) (Cunningham 2005). The uniqueness of the individual woman is unimportant to obstetrics as the woman is seen as essentially disconnected from her uterus. The limited and limiting nature of the obstetric paradigm means that anything outside the three Ps is considered to have no impact on the birthing process. The obstetric paradigm ignores the impact of the woman's thoughts and emotions on her physiology and on her baby. The impact that the physical, spiritual and psychodynamic environment has on women and babies is also ignored and denied by the obstetric paradigm.

In recent years, the importance of the birth environment has been recognised (Lepori 1994; NCT 2003; Walsh 2006a,b) but this book is the first to describe, explain and predict the impact of environment on childbearing. We do this by reviewing a vast array of research and scholarly literature and by reflecting on our own lives as women and our practice as midwives.

Finally, we bring this knowledge together in a theoretically integrated way.

An underlying tenet of Birth Territory and Midwifery Guardianship is that women are diverse, individual, changing and embodied. The core of the theory is respect for the uniqueness of the individual woman and the moment to moment relationships she forms with her ever-changing environment and the impact of this on her birth physiology, experience and outcomes. Our midwifery theory draws from and contributes to biological, architectural, psychological, sociological, post-structural and feminist theory.

If you are a woman who is pregnant or considering pregnancy, we invite you to use this book in any way that helps you to feel stronger and surer about what you want for the birth of your baby and beyond. If you are a midwife, you are an integral part of the environment for childbearing women. This book proposes a role for the midwife as the guardian of the birth territory. As midwives, researchers and writers, we value and have a preference for normal birth. However, we acknowledge that each birth is an individual journey and there are times when intervention is appropriate. Indeed, midwives need to do everything in their power to support and enhance the woman's positive sense of self and connection with her unborn and newborn baby, regardless of how the pregnancy, labour and birth progresses.

Chapter 1 introduces some theories that will allow you to begin the process of understanding how power operates. This understanding is necessary because no 'birth territory' can exist outside the gendered, political, economic, social and legal networks of power within a given culture. These networks are continuously acting consciously and unconsciously on women, midwives and doctors in ways that limit and direct what is possible in terms of birth territories at the local level. At the social level, the networks of power have the effect of reproducing medical domination whilst simultaneously inducing the submission of women and midwives. Feeling submissive actually weakens people physically, intellectually and emotionally. We argue that women need to feel strong and confident to make the best decisions for themselves and their babies.

Chapter 2 describes a theory of 'Birth Territory'. A review of the literature shows a paucity of theory or research on the effect of environment on birthing. The theory of birth territory challenges the dominant medical theory of birth which views women's bodies as if they were unreliable machines. Three contrasting birth stories are used to illustrate the theory. Key elements of the environment that appear to have an effect on birthing outcomes are identified and discussed. The first story is a brief description of a birth in a contemporary Australian delivery suite. Next there is a description of the labour and birth of Lapis, a female monkey. The third story is of a woman, Barbara, in a home birth environment. The final section of the chapter concerns the theoretical development of 'Birth Territory' with the concepts physical terrain, jurisdiction and midwifery guardianship.

The third chapter focuses on Midwifery Guardianship of the Birth Territory which involves working with the spirituality of birth. Midwifery guardianship is a form of spiritual practice which involves controlling who crosses the boundaries of the birth space while creating and maintaining a sacred harmony within that space. A 'midwifery guardian' is spiritually aware and supports the woman to quieten her rational, judging, thinking mind so that she may enter a non-ordinary state of consciousness: the ideal state for giving birth. The midwife guardian encourages the woman's mindfulness within the non-ordinary state which includes the woman focusing on welcoming the birth of her baby while sensing and responding to her body signals. By providing an environment in which the woman can trust and work with her own body, the midwife guardian supports the woman as she gains access to her 'inner self' and 'inner power' which is necessary if the woman is to give birth using her own power. Accessing the 'inner self' also allows a woman to deal with unanticipated complications without fear and to be able to choose the best options for herself and her baby. The chapter concludes by discussing the ethics of working with women when they are extraordinarily vulnerable during birthing from within a non-ordinary consciousness state.

The fourth chapter considers the environment in terms of women's transformation during childbearing and the impact on women's sense of themselves as integrated and whole 'embodied selves'. Women's social and personal transformations during childbirth are explored by contrasting socially sanctioned rituals (including medicalized childbirth) and the personally developed rituals (including movement in labour) that women make for themselves when they are in a supportive environment. The Western over-reliance on rational thinking is shown to misrepresent how medical birth and natural birth are interpreted; this leads women and midwives to the use of socially sanctioned rituals even when natural birth is the stated intention. The integrating power and knowledge of 'non-rationality' (incorporating feelings and intuitions) are identified as resources that profoundly affect outcomes during the experiential reality of childbirth change. Women change throughout the childbearing year by a series of intimate ongoing cycles of change. When these are respected by everyone in her environment, then a woman's potential during childbirth moves beyond the habitually chosen practices of socially sanctioned rituals. The chapter introduces a portion of the theory 'Territories of the Self' and gives definition to terms such as 'embodied self', 'spirit' and 'soul', while discussing the boundaries of potential. An awareness of the 'Territories of the Self' enables spiritual practices during childbirth by both woman and midwife. These practices can guide us towards the actualization of the woman's potential. Unique spiritual practices teach both woman and midwives to value and maintain a sense of integrated wholeness during the ongoing changes of childbirth and of life. The theory is illustrated by stories that were constructed during in-depth, sequential interviews with 14 women who were having their first babies.

Chapter 5 examines the complex interplay of hormonal influences on the physiology of birth and the role that environment has in either optimizing or interfering with normal physiology. Evidence from animal and human research shows that the environment for birth affects which of two possible states of being predominate in birth; the woman will either be calm and relaxed through a hormonally mediated connection to others or suffer a disconnected state of heightened anxiety and fear. Fearful emotional states disrupt secretion of the hormone, Oxytocin, which is central for effective uterine activity in labour and also for a wide range of behaviours designed to ensure that women and their babies are attached to each other and love grows. Evidence from the nature/nurture debate presented in the chapter leads to a deeper understanding of the potential lifelong consequences of disruptions to the normal physiology of childbirth. This reveals how the environment for birth needs to be shaped and protected by the midwife so that normal birth can take place.

Chapter 6 reveals the critical importance of the prenatal and perinatal period in laying the spiritual, emotional and physical framework for the developing person. The role of pre-conceptual health and nutrition of both parents in genetic expression is emphasized. How the spiritual, emotional and physical wellbeing of both parents before and during pregnancy affects their growing baby is explained. Insights into prenatal psychodynamic and emotional development demonstrate that the unborn baby functions like a tape recorder and subjectively records its mother's thoughts and feelings as its own. The unborn baby lays down imprints of patterns of thinking, feeling and behaviour to form the blueprint from which its life will be built. Depending upon the spiritual, emotional and physical health of the woman and the environment in which she lives, the prenatal environment of the baby can be experienced as loving and blissful or a source of terror, anxiety and a sense of hopelessness, with lifelong consequences for the individual.

Chapter 7 examines what the authors refer to as mindbodyspirit architecture for birth. The moving, feeling, dreaming body of the birthing woman and her requirements for an optimal birth environment are articulated. This chapter provides a detailed list of the elements in the geography, architecture and metaphysics of birth spaces to which women will consciously and unconsciously respond. The new architecture assists with integrating the left and right hemispheres of the brain leading to an integrated and 'best of both worlds' birthing space. One of the authors is an architect experienced in the design of birth spaces. The midwife authors provide several illustrated examples of mindbodyspirit birth architecture from their midwifery practice.

Chapter 8 describes some of the problems that have prevented midwives from being effective and sensitive. The characteristics of what is called 'The New Midwifery' and its relevance to what is a critical period in human life is discussed. The basic argument of this chapter is that organizations in which midwives practice should enable the creation of the new midwifery, but the majority of maternity services make it very difficult to practise effectively. The result is that birthing environments are less than optimal. Drawing on theory, evidence and experience the chapter proposes ways of making the maternity services better for midwives, in order that they may support women and their families to have the best births possible in their particular circumstances.

In Chapter 9, Michel Odent argues that there is an unstable relationship between obstetricians, midwives and other caregivers because the basic needs of labouring women and newborn babies should, but seldom do, take priority. The labouring woman needs to feel secure, without feeling observed, in a warm enough place, and to be protected against any sort of disruptive left-brain stimulation (language,

light, lack of privacy, being aware of a possible danger, etc). The chapter provides an historical overview of how the birth territory came to be the domain of the obstetrician. It discusses how newly developing specialties such as sonography, fetal medicine, obstetric anaesthesiology, neonatology, perinatology, epidemiology, and genetic counselling encroach on both the obstetrician's sense of his territory and the birth territory of women and babies.

Chapter 10 examines philosophical, organizational and cultural change strategies used to successfully implement woman-centred birth territory within publicly funded maternity services in Western countries. The authors use examples from their experiences of improving the quality of birthing territory for women and midwives in Australia and the United Kingdom. They discuss the role of leadership in facilitating change and the value of collaborative relationships in enabling optimum experiences for women and their families.

The way we think about and provide services which manage childbirth can create feelings of either love or fear. The obstetric paradigm, which is based on risk identification and early intervention, is a fear-based paradigm. Throughout this book, the authors demonstrate the importance of providing a loving, nurturing environment so that the holistic health of women and babies is optimized during pregnancy, birth and beyond. The following poem by Michael Leunig expresses the differences between the authors' approach to Birth Territories and Midwifery Guardianship and that of the standard Western obstetric paradigm that currently controls maternity services. In so many situations, it is fear that is responsible for creating the unnecessary interventions and complications that are so common in modern childbearing.

Love and Fear
There are only two feelings.
Love and fear
There are only two languages.
Love and fear
There are only two activities.
Love and fear
There are only two motives,
two procedures, two frameworks,
two results.
Love and fear.
Love and fear.
(Leunig 1990, A Common Prayer: A cartoonist talks to God. Harper Collins, Sydney. Reprinted with permission.)

Kathleen Fahy
Maralyn Foureur
Carolyn Hastie

Newcastle, 2008

References

Cumingham G (ed) 2005 Williams Obstetrics, New York. McGraw Hill.

Lepori B 1994 Freedom of movement in birth places. Children's environments 11(2): 81–87.

Leunig M 1990 A Common Prayer: A cartoonist talks to God. Harper Collins Publishers, Sydney.

National Childbirth Trust 2003 Improving the built environment and culture for birth. NCT, London.

Walsh D 2006a Nesting and matrescence as distinctive features of a free-standing birth centre. Midwifery 22(3): 228–239.

Walsh D 2006b Subverting the assembly-line: childbirth in a free-standing birth centre. Social Science and Medicine 62(6): 1330–1336.

Acknowledgements

This book was inspired by the presentations and sharing of ideas at the first 'Keeping Birth Normal' conference held in New Zealand at Victoria University of Wellington in 2004 where Maralyn Foureur, Kathleen Fahy and Carolyn Hastie were all contributors. The conference motivated the establishment of a Normal Birth Research Unit at the university as well as started international, cross disciplinary conversations about gathering together key ideas that focus on 'Keeping Birth Normal' in a book such as this.

We wish to acknowledge the contributions of our brilliant colleagues whose work the book contains and thank them for their stimulating ideas and wisdom as well as their commitment to the project over the many years of gestation.

We are indebted to the incredibly important contributions made in both known and unknown ways by the women and their families with whom we have worked during careers spanning 30 years in midwifery, academe and research. Being with women throughout their childbearing experience has provided, and continues to provide, a profound learning and enriching opportunity.

Kathleen Fahy:
I acknowledge my greatest teachers first: my mother, Daphne, and daughters Jyai and Lauren. I acknowledge some primary sources of my own personal and spiritual development which has been profoundly influenced by Stan Grof's theories and practices concerning transpersonal transformation and ideas arising from Tibetan Buddhism. I wish to acknowledge Ms Jenny Parratt for the shared genesis of the initial ideas that formed the foundation for early theorising about the impact of birth territory on birthing women. Ms Carolyn Hastie has been a personal friend and clinical mentor; from her I have learned the type of midwifery that is explored in this book. It is my hope that others will be inspired, by our book, to practise as midwifery guardians.

Maralyn Foureur:
When I became a midwife I asked my mother how I had been born. 'Childbirth without Fear' by Grantley Dick Read had recently been published and she read it from cover to cover in an effort to dispel her anxiety about what was about to unfold. When labour started and the pains became stronger, she practised the recommended breathing and went to hospital. My father was left in the waiting room and my mother was wheeled into a delivery room, laid up on a narrow bed and was left alone. When the 'matron' later saw her pattered breathing she was admonished to 'stop that nonsense' so my mother stuffed her handkerchief into her mouth to stop from crying out. Many hours later she had a mask placed over her nose and mouth and chloroform was dripped onto it until she was no longer aware of what was happening and I was born. I acknowledge my strong and beautiful mother for enduring such an experience and still loving me. I also acknowledge and thank my two children, Cleo and Heath whose births gave me the confidence and embodied knowing of how empowering the experience of becoming a mother can be. Their births ignited a passionate interest in me for ensuring that childbearing women are respected and nurtured so that they can grow their babies and give birth in optimal environments. Very recently my daughter invited me to be present as she gave birth to her first child. What a treasured gift!

Now I am a grandmother to two beautiful granddaughters, Ollie and Morgan and I am working to ensure they have an opportunity to know the same power in their experiences of childbirth - a long time in the future. I hope this book contributes in some way.

Carolyn Hastie:
I want to acknowledge my mother, who taught me the primal importance of a deep, loving connection with our family of origin and especially our mothers; my beautiful and precious children Julia, Ben, Jack and Edward, my biggest teachers, who taught me the importance of being clear, relaxed, loving and consistent; my treasured friends, colleagues and students who have taught me the value of having an open, willing curiosity. I acknowledge Frederick Leboyer, whose book "Birth without Violence" opened my eyes to the amazing abilities of the newborn and our ethical and practical responsibilities as midwives in facilitating a loving space to welcome newborn babies. Ina May Gaskin in her book "Spiritual Midwifery" introduced me to the whole woman who gives birth, replacing the prevailing construct, common at that time, of a physical female body that is mechanically 'delivered' of an infant. I want to acknowledge Anne Saxton, my Service Manager, and Dr Andrew Bisits, my Director of Obstetrics, who are ardent advocates for keeping birth normal and women centred maternity services. I hope Anne, Andrew and other visionaries like them, who see the value in keeping women at the centre of our considerations about maternity care, will find much to support their work in this book. I also wish to acknowledge my co-editors, Maralyn and Kathleen, dear friends and colleagues, without whom this book would not have been written. These women are great mentors, friends and thinkers. Finally, I want to acknowledge all the wonderful women, babies and families I have had the honour of supporting through childbirth, who have taught and continue to teach me how to be 'present' to and support them in their reality and their process.

December 2007

Section 1

Theories and practices

Chapter 1

Power and the social construction of birth territory

Kathleen Fahy

No birth territory can exist outside the gendered, political, economic, social and legal power networks of a given culture. These networks are continuously acting consciously and unconsciously on women, midwives and doctors in ways that limit and direct what is possible in terms of birth territories at the local level. At the social level, the networks of power have the effect of reproducing medical domination and simultaneously the submission of women and midwives within whole cultures. I would argue that feeling submissive actually weakens people physically, intellectually and emotionally. Women need to feel strong and confident in order to birth using their own power and in order to make the best decisions for themselves and their babies. This chapter introduces some important theoretical ideas that will help you to understand how power operates at the social and the individual level. The story below is an example of networks of power in operation in contemporary Western society. The story also shows that the individual is not powerless; indeed it tells of one woman's creative use of her own power.

Madeleine's story

When Madeleine Bray was pregnant after her first child was born by caesarean section, she repeatedly tried to negotiate an agreement with doctors at the Royal Brisbane Hospital (RBH) to have an active labour. The RBH doctors had said that Madeleine would be required to lie down throughout labour,

Madeleine's story   Continued

have a fetal heart rate monitor attached and a cannula in her vein. The doctors had booked a caesarean section for her 'just in case'. Because of their refusal to allow her to labour in the way she wanted she inquired at another hospital if she could be more active in birthing. That hospital agreed. Knowing that she could have the kind of birth she wanted at another hospital, Madeleine cancelled the caesarean section that was scheduled for her at RBH without giving an explanation. When the RBH obstetric division (note, the actual doctor remained invisible) realized that the caesarean had been cancelled by Madeleine, they (he) no doubt thought she was going to have a home birth. They reported Madeleine to the hospital administrators who in turn reported her to the Child Protection agency for child abuse or neglect. Madeleine was visited at her home by child protection officers at a time when she was in the early stages of labour. Madeleine went on to have a natural birth and a healthy baby at the second hospital (Wenham 2005).

This story caused a storm of protests about women's rights to choose how and where they birth. That Madeleine is a woman is important; there are no newspaper reports of men being required to undergo medical treatments against their wills. The story also demonstrates that medical power is supported politically by the State. The hidden rule, revealed by Madeleine's resistance, is that if a woman wants to access a hospital as a place to give birth, she must submit to medical control. If a woman seeks to avoid the medical system entirely, as health officials no doubt thought Madeleine Bray was trying to do, a single phone call to an arm of government will result in her privacy being invaded and the possible loss of her baby to the welfare system. The story implies that a staff member from the maternity unit made that call on the behest of the obstetrician; it was possibly even a midwife who picked up the phone to report Madeleine Bray. The uneasy relationship between obstetrics and midwifery will be analysed and deconstructed in this chapter and in the following chapters. From where does medicine derive so much power over women, birth and midwifery?

DEFINING SOME KEY POSTMODERN TERMS

Before proceeding to the next section I draw the reader's attention to some simplified definitions of key postmodern theoretical terms included in the Glossary at the end of the book. Where the key term is also described in the text the first time the word is used it is follow with an asterisk (*) and the references are given within the text. Some would argue that I shouldn't provide simple meanings for terms that are used in multiple different ways by different theorists and even by the same theorist at different times. Notwithstanding the value of such an argument I have decided to provide these definitions as a beginning so that someone new to the field of postmodern theory will have a place to begin.

FOUCAULT AND POWER

Michel Foucault made a life-time study of power and the socio-historical context. He explored the ways in which certain groups exercised more power while other groups exercised less power. He produced a number of insights that were quite profoundly new at the time (1970–1980s). Foucault's concept of power* challenges the dominant view which sees that a limited number of people 'have power' which is used repressively against a much larger number of people who are 'without power'. He wrote in Power/Knowledge (Foucault 1980) that power is:

> 'never in anybody's hands, never appropriated as a commodity or piece of wealth. Power is employed and exercised through a net-like organization. And not only do individuals circulate between its threads; they are always in the position of simultaneously undergoing and exercising this power.' (p. 98)

A critical insight of Foucault was his recognition of the inseparability of power and knowledge (1980). He argued that individuals and groups have knowledges that are expressed as discourses*. Discourses of knowledge, because they are the basis of power, always contested by groups that seek to exercise more power.

POSTMODERNISM, METANARRATIVES AND DISCOURSES

Foucault has been considered a postmodern* theorist. Lyotard (1984) cogently defined a postmodernist as one who had an attitude of incredulity towards metanarratives*. Metanarratives from a postmodernist perspective are myths that over-simplify and blind us to subtleties, complexity and exceptions (Lyotard 1984). In line with the postmodern rejection of metanarratives, dis-courses* too are neither true nor false (Lupton 1992; Traynor 2003). 'Truth' is socially constructed in that some discourses get to be accepted as 'true' while others are marginalized within soci-ety. Social norms are embedded in dominant discourses which then exercise normalising influ-ence on subjects; i.e. we behave as we are expected to behave (Foucault 1979).

POWER/KNOWLEDGE

Foucault's (1980) concept of knowledge/power is written like this to demonstrate the insepara-bility of power and knowledge. He argued that power and knowledge are self-referential and synergistic. This means that having the public accept the discipline's knowledge claims as 'true' has the effect of increasing the power of the dis-cipline. It is critical to be aware that it is society that decides which knowledge and authority it will accept and which it will marginalize. Thus, society privileges certain discourses and certain groups, e.g. obstetric discourse and obstetri-cians while simultaneously marginalizing nor-mal birth discourses, women's self-knowledge and midwifery knowledge.

DISCIPLINARY POWER

Foucault was concerned about the rise of profes-sional power; particularly medical power and how that power operated within social institu-tions e.g. hospitals. Doctors, he claimed, used a form of coercive power that he named 'disciplin-ary power'* (Foucault 1979). Disciplinary power, Foucault argues, operates concurrently with, and may subvert, the subject's legal power. (Foucault 1980). In contrast to the way is which legal power operates, openly and clearly, disciplinary power seeks invisibility. Unlike legal power, disciplin-ary power requires the co-operation of the sub-ject. Disciplinary power is difficult to detect, usually not becoming visible until the object of disciplinary power offers resistance (Foucault 1982). The subtle ways in which the subject's co-operation is gained are important to understand

because this unmasks the attempt to use power invisibly. We can even use power in ways that are invisible to ourselves. For example, midwives often don't know that they are acting coercively because, using unconscious defence mechanisms, they are not aware that they are being coercive until a woman resists or complains.

Surveillance, the gaze

The disciplines derive much of their power from putting the subjects on display, while those who are controlling the situation remain unseen. Foucault (1979) used the idea of the Panopticon (observational tower in the octagonal shaped jail) as a model to facilitate understanding of how surveillance is central to the operation of disciplinary power. Surveillance* depends upon what Foucault called 'the gaze'. Gazing affects us all as social subjects. We are usually on dis-play and even if not consciously on display we are usually aware that someone may be watching us or monitoring our movements. Because of this we moderate our own behaviour in line with dominant norms. Thus we usually become docile and obedient subjects who police ourselves in relation to the internalized expectations of the dominant groups in society (Foucault 1979). For feminist this generalized 'gaze' is male. Sandra Bartky (1988) wrote:

'Disciplinary power is peculiarly modern: it does not rely upon violent or public sanctions, nor does it seek to restrain the freedom of the female body to move from place to place [but there is] regulation that is perpetual and exhaustive – a regulation of the body's size and contours, its appetite, posture, gestures and general comportment in space, and the appearance of each of its visible parts.' (p. 80)

For feminists, the gaze is thought to be male even when women do the gazing. Women know and understand the dominant male fantasies (discourses) about how women should look and behave and thus women police each other in relation to male expectations.

This gaze of medical surveillance is a pre-requisite for medical power. The subjects of medical power must make their bodies open to the medical gaze. Patients give up their bodily secrets in the belief that medical power can control disease. Medical knowledge has been, and continues to be, dependent upon gazing on and inside patients (alive and dead). In maternity services medical gazing occurs, for example, when women come to hospital for antenatal care and are subjected to antenatal surveillance. In the birthing suite medical power is intensified by the use of cardiotocographs. Further, in most delivery suites doctors walk into the rooms of labouring women to check on how they are progressing against medically defined norms for each stage of labour. Midwives who are employed in hospitals are legally required to be complicit in medical gazing by surveillance of, and reporting on, the women.

Docility: reward and punish

Disciplines, Foucault said, induce submission by promising people rewards for compliance and punishments for non-compliance; this is normally done implicitly (1984). When this idea is applied to medicine, the promises that medicine offers are 'life', 'health' and 'pain relief', while the punishments are fears of 'pain', 'death' or 'disability'.

Both midwives and women are usually docile in relation to medical power/knowledge. There are many rewards and punishments built into the education and training as midwives, (many of whom were first trained in the medical model via nursing). The punishments for not behaving as 'docile' subjects within the health care system are well known and include being shunned, criticized and ostracized by one's colleagues, in addition to being subject to formal administrative sanctions (Huard and Fahy 1999). Another reason midwives behave submissively is to avoid responsibility. One of the most potent pleasures is to let go of responsibility and hand over decision-making to the powerful other. This frees us from the worry and anxiety of taking control of the situation and being held accountable (Foucault 1980). Not wanting to feel or be held accountable helps to explain why some midwives actively resist the introduction of midwifery models.

Some of the reasons that pregnant women make themselves docile towards obstetricians have been implied above; i.e. being seen as a 'nice woman' who is not wilful. Taking this position avoids the risk of the woman being shunned at a time of great need and vulnerability. Her deepest fear is that she will not get help, care and support when she needs it during birth. Also, being docile brings with it the relief of handing over of responsibility for childbirth and its outcome. In this way the woman does not hold herself accountable and will not be held accountable by her significant others.

Taking Foucault's ideas into account I define 'Power' as energy which enables an individual (or a group) to be able to do or obtain what they want (Northrup 1998). Power is essential for living; without it we would not move at all. Power is ethically neutral; this is consistent with Foucault's notion of power which he argued was productive; not necessarily oppressive (Foucault 1980).

This section on Foucault has shown that if women want to be in control of their birth space with midwives acting as protectors and guardians then this is threatening to medical power. In the section to follow I summarize the process by which medicine originally subordinated midwifery. The main reason for doing this is to examine the contextual similarities and difference between now and then. This knowledge helps us to recognize the power strategies that are currently being used by medicine. Such knowledge is necessary in planning how these strategies might be subverted or countered by contemporary women and midwives when seeking to promote birth territories that are most likely to support women to birth their babies.

MEDICINE AND THE CONTROL OF BIRTH TERRITORY

I recently published a paper on an Australian history of the subordination of midwifery in the journal, Women and Birth (Fahy 2007). That paper summarizes the history of the decline of midwifery and the rise of obstetrics in Europe and the United Kingdom. This acts as the broader context for understanding the subordination of midwifery in Australia which is an example of the application of a Western meta-narrative. Medicine in the late 19th and early 20th century was composed almost entirely of men who shared the same power base as other dominant males; they were white, well educated and from economically richer families. It was these males who owned or managed every institution of society; the army, the church, the law, the newspapers, the government etc. These privileges, combined with an informal brotherhood of dominant men created a powerful base for the success of the medical campaign to subordinate midwifery.

At the start of their campaign against midwives medicine has some legal power on its side. The Medical Registration Act of 1858 was the first expression of medical legal power; it limited who could practise medicine and allowed medicine to control their own education and registration (Arnold 2001). From their perspective the act didn't go far enough as it did not sanction the legal takeover of midwives. Disciplinary power, therefore, was the major form of power that medicine used at this time. The medical campaign against midwives exploited educational, class and gender differences to stigmatize midwives as unsafe practitioners (Willis 1983). Hospitals were being built in all major large numbers during the same time as this struggle was occurring, i.e. late 19th century and early 20th century. Hospitals were environments where nurses were employed and medicine reigned supreme. Unlike midwives, who were independent women living in the community; nurses followed the Nightingale model which ensured that they followed doctors' orders (1980). Hospitals, therefore, were ideal places for childbearing women to be brought under medical surveillance. The government wanted to retain and educate midwives but in spite of government pleading nurses aligned with doctors and refused to teach the lay midwives (Willis 1983; Summers 1999). The refusal of medicine and nursing to respond educationally to their own espoused concerns about midwives being unsafe practitioners unmasks a real motivation of occupational takeover.

During their struggle to subordinate midwives medical men networked with each other and with other dominant men. These men included politician, judges, lawyers, newspaper owners and capitalists (Willis 1983). Thus, the social leaders believed their medical friends and they propagated the false belief that midwives caused childbirth fever. Then, as now, powerful change normally happen when first the powerful elite and then the middle class adopt a new idea. All of this was being driven by medical disciplinary power which required

ongoing effort. But, with the support of governments disciplinary power was eventually converted into legal power so no further effort was required to suppress midwives.

Following a Royal Commission into the declining birth rate (1904) the government introduced a baby bonus of five pounds in 1912 (Willis 1983). Medicine was a major beneficiary of the baby bonus in that the payment of the money was legally restricted to women who had medically supervised births. The medical registration act eventually did form the foundation for medicine to be able to claim an ever increasing occupational territory and the domination of all other health disciplines (Willis 1983). Other laws also converted medical disciplinary power to legal power including the Private Hospitals Acts (which were proclaimed in different states on different dates in the 1920s). The Private Hospitals Act gave the department of health power to regulate and accredit the lying-in cottages run by midwives. Since the departments of health were and are advised primarily by doctors this act gave indirect power to doctors over midwives in private practice; their chief occupational competitor (Adcock et al 1986; Graf-Smith 2003). The Nurses Registration Acts were also proclaimed at about that time. Doctors continued to chair the Nurses Registration Boards in all states until the second half of the 20th century which is a demonstration of their ongoing domination.

Medicine and the state in contemporary society
The relations between medicine and the State were and are crucial to the way in which health care is designed, funded and delivered. In contemporary society the State in Western countries is capitalist* in nature. In order for capitalist economies to succeed the State must promote and protect capital accumulation i.e. wealth creation. The State must create and enforce laws that keep society stable and ensure the smooth functioning of business. Governments need to ensure an adequate supply of workers, including importing them if needed. Governments are also responsible for educating the workers of tomorrow; for keeping workers healthy and if sick, for returning them to health if possible. These latter roles are a point of intersection

between the interests of capitalists, doctors and the State (Willis 1983).

Evan Willis, writing recently, argues that medical power has decreased from its high point in about 1970. More and more we talk of 'health' and health workers and not so much medicine and medical workers (Willis 2006). Support for medicine is still expressed, however, through government initiated law, policy and actions. Government actions that benefit medical interests occur daily and are usually mediated by the recommendations emanating from health related committees. Both federal and state governments place doctors, in dominant numbers and in chairing roles on the vast majority of committees that plan and manage health services, including maternity care. Some committees have one or two midwives and possibly a consumer. The committee chairs are invariably medical therefore the outcomes of the committees usually have a heavy weighting towards medical interests. This committee composition is replicated at the health service level. Thus, policy and planning related to maternity services occur by committee where the composition of each committee is usually weighted towards medicine.

A major role for the State is the legitimation of the discourses, or knowledge claims, of the dominant class (Wills, p. 28). Helping dominant groups have their ideological claims accepted as 'true' also helps governments to stay in power. That is in part because it keeps the dominate males in society happy and positive about the government and in part because legitimating the dominant discourses sometimes serve State interests. A convergence of interests occurs, for example, if the dominant discourses can be used with voters in a way that demonstrates support for government policy. Thus, for example, doctors and governments insist that what needs to happen to make indigenous women safe in birth is to take them out of their homelands and make them travel and live in a major city to await medically supervised birth. Even though doctors can produce no research evidence to support this, their claim is believed and enforced by government; no doubt in part because it is cheaper than providing birthing on the homelands as the indigenous women want. The Midwifery discourse, that well women with straight forward pregnancies can

have their births safely on the homelands, is marginalized. This happens even when there is evidence of safe and satisfying birthing in remote locations as is happening for the indigenous women at the Innulitsivik Birthing Centre in Puvirnituq in northern Canada (Tookalak 2000).

The social and educational advances of women and midwives have levelled the occupational playing field to some extent. Today, in the context of an Australia-wide shortage of obstetricians and GP obstetricians, governments are motivated to provide maternity services close to where the voters live. Thus there is a synergy of interests between maternity consumers, midwives and government. For example, in the state of New South Wales, the government is extending midwifery-led models of care; including free standing birthing centres and publicly funded homebirth. This is an example of midwives and women building networks, finding support and using power to bring about desired changes to maternity services.

I argued, above, that all government departments and the State as a whole protect the interests of the dominant class; i.e. to create and build wealth (Willis 1983, pp. 26–27). However, the State should not be viewed as a unified entity but as a set of power relations between groups with conflicting and competing ideologies. Each of the arms of government is composed of a hierarchically organized bureaucracy; thus the Department of Health, the hospitals and the departments within hospitals. The State bureaucracy is largely populated with workers who have a working class ideology who are seeking to change society for the better of the working class and the poor. The business of government involves bringing parties with competing interest together; the outcomes of such exchanges are not completely predictable (Willis 1983).

Speaking generally of the current time, medicine has changed and so has the broader society. Because higher education now has no up front fees we have seen a much more diverse range of doctors who now come from both sexes, all classes and all races. Women are now better educated and more powerful than they were. Nurses and midwives are all now university educated and much more engaged in public debate about health care. Midwives and women are actively challenging anti-midwife ideology by countering with research evidence via professional journals. The whole evidence-based medicine movement has had an effect of limiting the powers of individual doctors by challenging them to provide evidence for their treatments. Midwives and women are asking for woman-centred birthing and they are being heard on radio, television and read in the newspapers. They are being consulted by governments; something that was unheard of in the 1880s. These social factors have increased power for women and midwives and led to diminution of dominant white male privilege that supported medicine in the past.

CONCLUSIONS

The idea of Birth Territory and Midwifery Guardianship challenges the medical control of birth which they fought so hard to achieve. Practising midwifery in this way involves a level of independence which would likely encourage other dominated health disciplines to seek similar independence. Medicine as a whole, not just obstetrics, can be predicted to resist because of the broader threat to medical power.

Medical domination of midwifery and birth is diminishing or under serious challenge in most Western countries. Science is no longer the domain of a privileged few but can be conducted, read and critiqued by many. The State health departments know of the safety, satisfaction and cost-effectiveness of midwifery-led care. Midwives and women are asking for woman centred birthing and they are being heard on radio and television and read in the newspapers. A shortage of obstetricians and GP-obstetricians means that governments are motivated to provide maternity services close to where the voters live. Thus there is a synergy of interests between maternity consumers, midwives and government. In the state of New South Wales, Australia, at the time of writing the government has committed to extending midwifery-led models of care; including publicly funded homebirth.

QUESTIONS FOR DISCUSSION

1. What are the differences between legal and disciplinary power?
2. Under what circumstances does disciplinary power, which is usually not visible, become obvious?
3. What are the punishments and rewards that keep childbearing women docile in relation to the obstetric control of birth?
4. What effect does surveillance have on subjects?
5. Give examples of how employed midwives are subject to both legal and disciplinary power that makes them an arm of medical surveillance?
6. Using Foucault's ideas explain the relations between hospitals as institutions and medical power/knowledge.
7. How different are contemporary Western metanarratives from those of 100 years ago?
8. Why were medicine's historical efforts to professionalize so successful and nursing's were so limited?
9. Medicine's historical claim that midwives were the cause of puerperal sepsis was wrong and there was evidence to implicate doctors instead. What were the sources of power that allowed medicine's anti-midwife discourse to become the dominant legitimated one?
10. To what extent has modern medicine expanded its disease model beyond individual pathology and single causes?
11. Are Western countries patriarchal in nature: why or why not?
12. How are relations of power between midwifery and medicine both different from and similar to what they were 100 years ago?

References

Adcock WU, Bayliss et al 1984 With curage and devotion. Anvil Press for the NSW Midwives Association, Marrickville.

Arnold P 2001 Professional regulation. The Oxford companion to medicine. S Lock, J Last and G Dunea. Oxford, Oxford Reference Online, 2006.

Bartky SL 1988 Foucault, femininity, and the modernization of patriarchal power. Feminism and Foucault. Reflections on resistance. I Diamond and L Quinby. Northeastern University Press, Boston, pp. 61–86.

Butler J 1994 Feminism as radical humanism. Allen and Unwin, Sydney.

Fahy K 2007 An Australian history of the medical subordination of midwifery. Women and Birth 20: 1.

Foucault M 1979 Discipline and punish: the birth of the prison. Vintage Books, New York.

Foucault M 1980 Power/knowledge: selected interviews. Pantheon, New York.

Foucault M 1982 The subject and power. Michel Foucault: Beyond structuralism and hermeneutics. H Dreyfus and P Rabinow. Wheatsheaf, New York, Harvester, pp. 206–226.

Foucault M 1984 Introduction. The Foucault reader: An introduction to Foucault's thought. P Rabinow. New York, Pantheon, pp. 3–29.

Gaff-Smith M 2003 Midwives of the black soil plains. Triple D books, Wagga Wagga.

Huard, D. and Fahy K. 1999 Moral Distress, Advocacy and Burnout: Theorising the Links. International Journal of Nursing Practice. 5(1): 8–13.

Johnson P 1994 Feminism as radical humanism. Sydney, Allen and Unwin.

Lupton D 1992 Discourse analysis: a new methodology for understanding ideologies of health and illness. Australian Journal of Public Health 16(2): 145–149.

Lyotard JF 1984 The postmodern condition. Manchester University Press, Manchester.

Nightingale F 1980 Notes on nursing: What it is and what it is not. Churchill Livingstone, Edinburgh.

Northup, C. 1998 Women's bodies, Women's wisdom. Bath, Paitkus.

Rabinow P Ed 1984 The Foucault reader. Pantheon, New York.

Summers A 1999 The lost voice of midwifery. Collegian 5(3): 16–22.

Tookalak N 2000 The Innulitsivik Birthing Centre. Birth Place Magazine.

Traynor M 2003 Discourse analysis: ideology and professional practice. Advanced Qualitative Research for Nursing. J. Latimer. Oxford, Blackwell Publishing: 137–154.

Wenham M 2005 Labour of love. The Courier-Mail, Brisbane: 33.

Willis E 1983 Medical dominance: The division of labour in Australian health care. Allen & Unwin, Sydney.

Willis E 2006 Introduction: taking stock of medical dominance. Health Sociology Review 15(5): 421–430.

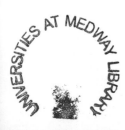

Chapter 2

Theorising birth territory

Kathleen Fahy

I am writing the beginning of this chapter while I am in a Yoga ashram which I will describe in detail, because many would say that this is an ideal environment for promoting health. Set in a bush land, the ashram is quiet, simple, uncluttered and peaceful. The ashram is populated with about 40 gentle people with whom I feel confident and safe. As we chop vegetables in the kitchen as part of Karma (work) Yoga we sing together and I feel a quiet joy. The whole environment supports me to let go of the need to organize and control things outside of myself. I naturally find myself living in the present: I am not worried about the future, nor do I cling to the past. Here I lie on the grass and look up through the leaves of the trees to the endless blue sky. I hear the different bird calls and the sound of leaves rustling in the wind. Time feels slowed down. I am usually so busy and so focused on matters that are my duty to attend to, but here my focus has turned towards myself. In this environment I notice things I would otherwise not, like the setting sun brightening one side of a cloud while the other side is the colour of midnight blue. I notice things inside myself that I might otherwise either not feel or, if felt, would ignore. I have written with some detail of the sanctuary of this place because I believe this is the type of environment that promotes inner focus which allows us to tune in to the subtle messages that our body and psyche send us. It is in this state, I have come to understand that our bodies and minds function at optimal levels of health, not just in birth, but at all times.

We have chosen to use the words 'birth terri-tory' rather than the word 'environment' since 'territory' encompasses the geographical and architectural boundaries of 'environment' but also includes notions of the people within a particular space and issues of power and control (Shorter Oxford English Dictionary 2002, p. 3220). The next chapter, concerning midwifery guardianship, pro-vides theory and clinical examples of how the woman's body–mind–spirit is holistically and irreducibly interconnected with the environment. This chapter focuses on the terrain of the birth environment. Some terminology may be new to readers; we have included some words in a glos-sary at the end of the book and these words are noted in this chapter with an asterisk (*).

The chapter begins with a summary of how feminism deals with notions of the biological body as a way of situating this theory within the broader postmodern* understanding of women as embodied* beings. Feminists are people who believe that the world and its people are domi-nated by patriarchy* and that patriarchy dis-advantages women. Next I sketch a few crucial aspects of the dominant medical metanarrative* that is supposed to explain birth. Then I present a review of the contemporary midwifery litera-ture concerning birth environment. This is done to demonstrate the paucity of theory or research on the effect of environment on birthing and thus demonstrate the need for this theory. Three con-trasting stories of births are examined here. The first is a brief description of a birth in a contempo-rary Australian delivery suite is presented as a way of demonstrating various aspects of the birth territory that have an effect on labour, birth and early mothering. The chapter then moves to a description of the labour and birth of Lapis, a female monkey, pregnant with her first baby, who gives birth in her natural setting. This description was chosen because it is really the only way to examine how a near-human primate gives birth without the intrusion of our human, techno-scientific culture into 'birth territory'. A birth story of a woman, Barbara, in a home birth environment completes the stories and shows how a birth sanctuary can be created in the home. Barbara's story has been analysed to identify key elements of the more natural environment that appear to have an effect on birthing outcomes.

The final section of the chapter concerns the theoretical development of birth territory with the concepts **physical terrain**, **jurisdiction** and **midwifery guardianship**. An ideal birth envi-ronment, I assert, is one in which the physical terrain more closely resembles the home and culture of the woman and one in which the woman feels safe, secure and in control of what happens to her and her baby.

An earlier version of some parts of this chapter were published with Jenny Parratt (Fahy and Parratt 2006). Jenny, Maralyn Foureur and Caro-lyn Hastie all contributed to the refinement of the theoretical concepts and responded to many drafts of the theory during its development.

FEMINISM AND THE BIOLOGICAL BODY

An assumption underpinning birth territory is that humans share similar birthing biology with other primates. Jenny Parratt and I presented some of these ideas at an interdisciplinary confer-ence where we were criticized by a feminist soci-ologist and labelled 'essentialist' for this belief. Other feminists in the room recoiled in horror and fear of being similarly labelled. 'Essentialist', in the context of this criticism, means that one thinks that all women are essentially the same because they share similar biology (Onions 2002); in our case it was even worse because we were saying women shared a similar biology to monkeys. I argue that we are not essentialist, but I do need to respond to the criticism because birth territory is too important a theory to allow it to be dismissed as simplistic 'essentialism'.

The so-called second wave feminists have argued that men and women are equal and that biology doesn't matter. Pregnancy and birth have been considered as a time of women's vulnerability and thus women were advised to limit childbear-ing and get over it quickly (Friedan 1963). These assumptions have served women well in the public domain where women have prospered. When 'equality' or 'liberal feminist' has been translated into law however, 'equality' has meant 'sameness'. This has resulted in some bizarre legal construc-tions; for example 'the American legal definition of pregnancy as a "disability" for the purpose of employment benefits (*California Federal* v. *Guerra*, Ninth Circuit, 1985)' (Mellor 2003).

Feminist theorists continue to be divided about how to deal with the material body, let alone the maternal body. The problem for the majority of feminists, including post-feminists like Naomi Wolf (1993), is that they leave the body out of their theorising. This has resulted in feminists trying to deal with the concept of 'women' without having to deal with the material bodies or their maternity. Birth territory theory is consistent with the position of the so called 'feminists of difference' who do explore female bodily experience (Irigaray 1985; Whitford 1991; Grosz 1994; Kristeva 1995; Young 2005). With them, I acknowledge the effect that the social environment has on the body and on behaviour, but I refuse to turn away from the biological body as a site of knowledge. Nor do I believe that all knowledge resides in knowing the body as medicine does. Indeed, I see the body as a site of knowing and remembering. Stanley and Wise (1993) caution against the type of criticism that Jenny and I encountered at the conference. Stanley and Wise claim that anti-essentialism is a form of dichotomous thinking which can be just as limiting as essentialism. In light of postmodernist* theories most feminists would now seek to be open to learning on both sides of the old dichotomies.

REVIEW OF RELATED LITERATURE

Taking a Foucauldian perspective (see Chapter 1) the theory of birth territory is a subjugated discourse with medicine having the dominant discourse. The medical discourse forms part of the broader dominant Western metanarrative which holds that science is superior to nature and that science and technology can be relied upon to solve human problems (Johnson 1994). For childbearing women this belief translates to the idea that obstetrics can manage birth better than women and babies. The obstetric discourse is based on a reductionistic belief that cause of any health-related phenomena, in this case birth, can be understood in a simplistic way; i.e. one 'cause' leading to another in a linear chain of 'causes'. For example, modern obstetrics explains labour and birth using a machine metaphor. The woman's uterus is termed 'the powers' which works something like a piston to push the baby down and out. The uterus is assumed to function separately from the woman's mind and emotions. Further, the baby is thought of as an inert package; the 'passenger' who passes passively through the maternal 'passages' on the way to being born. Because the environment operates holistically and on multiple levels all at once it cannot be accounted for in this linear, reductionistic medical model. In obstetrics the effect of environment is therefore not considered (Cunningham 2005).

A careful search of the midwifery literature found no explicit theory about the importance of environment on birth. For instance Gould (2002) asserts that the medicalized birth environment of the hospital acts subliminally to medicalize birth in the mind of the woman. Walsh (2000) writes about the negative impact of a 'bed birth' and argues for mobility in labour and removing the bed from centre stage. He later wrote about the different way in which the assembly line managerial model of hospital births is subverted by the privacy and distance of free-standing birth centres (Walsh 2006a). Further, he wrote about the importance of environment for women to feel safe and to be able to engage in nesting behaviours just like other mammals (Walsh 2006b).

There has been recent research on the impact of the environment on birth but this research is not explicitly guided by theory. A British study conducted by The National Childbirth Trust (NCT) (2003) evaluated women's experiences of their birth environment and their preferences for how they wanted the environment to be. Over half of the women who said each of the following factors were highly important did NOT have access to them when giving birth:

- Control over temperature.
- A pleasant place to walk.
- Sufficient pillows, floor mats and bean bags.
- A homely non-clinical environment.
- Not being overheard by others.
- Control over who came into the room.
- A place to get snacks and drinks.

Over one-third of the women who said each of the following factors were highly important did NOT have access to them when giving birth:

- A birth pool.
- A comfortable chair for companions.
- An en suite toilet, shower or bath, or easy access to these.
- Control over brightness of the light.

The recommendations from The NCT (2003) were therefore mostly about architectural design and interior decorating. Birth territory deals with the physical, the social and the metaphysical space and the issue of power concerning who is in control of the space; the totality of this is termed 'birth territory'. Further, the NCT research findings are not linked to any issues of birth outcomes; it is as if these environmental attributes are luxuries that do not confer any health benefits whereas in this book we are

arguing, in a number of ways, an important negative effect of medicalized environments and behaviours on birth.

Tara's story is presented below to demonstrate how the medical model of birth and the use of manipulative power (a form of disciplinary power) easily overwhelm the natural birth process. (See Chapter 1 for more details about power.) The unintended effect is that the very thing that medicine is trying to know, control and improve is actually damaged in the process.

TARA'S BIRTH IN A HOSPITAL BIRTH ENVIRONMENT

I observed this episode as a researcher when I was studying teenage transition to motherhood (Fahy 1995). A different analysis of this story was included in an earlier version of birth territory theory (Fahy and Parratt 2006).

Tara's story

Tara (19) was well known to me as a research participant. She was the daughter of a divorced woman who had a serious mental illness that required years of hospitalization. During those years Tara was sexually abused by three men who were supposed to be her carers. With my help she had devised a birth plan which included that if Tara felt she couldn't cope with the pain then she would have an epidural. In the description below I've italicized those phrases that are particularly relevant to the analysis of impact of environment on birthing. My notes at the time recorded my reflections.

At 06:00 hours, Tara had been labouring for about eight hours when she asked someone to telephone and request that I come in. The delivery suite was on the 3rd floor of the hospital. I walked straight into the room as *there was no door*, just a pink curtain partly covering the entrance. Tara was in a large, modern, *clinical-looking room*. All the furniture was *made of metal*. It had two windows but *the view was of another building*. The room was *air-conditioned*. The *lighting was by artificial* recessed fluorescent tubes. There was *a large, mobile operating theatre light* hanging over the bed. There was *oxygen and suction on the wall*.

A *baby resuscitation trolley* was 'hidden' behind a pink screen (although clearly visible to me). The bed was in the

centre of the room; its *end was facing the curtained doorway*. *Staff members entered the room uninvited and unannounced*. Tara was lying on her side on the bed, covered by a sheet. Her mother sat quietly beside her. Tara was awake and apparently relaxed. She had a working *epidural*, and an *electronic fetal monitor* was attached.

Shortly after I arrived the epidural wore off and Tara wanted it topped up. *Her request was refused* by the midwives who explained that as her cervix was fully dilated she wouldn't feel the urge to push and therefore a normal birth wouldn't be able to happen if she had a working epidural. Tara said she didn't care about a normal birth, she just wanted the epidural topped up but *the midwives wouldn't do what she wanted*.

After the refusal Tara became passive and sullen and continued to want the epidural topped up but she was not assertive in making this clear.

I urged her to speak up for herself which she did. Shortly afterwards *the senior medical registrar (whom Tara had never seen) came in and stood at the end of the bed* and said, with a degree of anger, 'we will top you up but you will probably need forceps now and that can damage the baby's head. You are a selfish girl who is putting her baby at risk'. Not waiting for a response,

---

Tara's story   Continued

he walked out and was never seen again. My assumption was that the midwives told the doctor and asked him to try to get Tara to desist from asking for an epidural top-up. Clearly she is being punished here; I felt I was being punished through Tara's additional suffering.

Tara turned her face away and without talking she cried softly. Except for crying she was essentially silent for the rest of the labour. Throughout the rest of the labour Tara was passive and sullenly compliant.

The epidural was finally topped up but only worked on one side so Tara continued to feel the pain fully on one side. After the episode with the doctor Tara's contractions became less frequent and much shorter. On medical orders the midwives began a Syntocinon infusion. Tara was given no further midwifery support. She was left for six hours in second stage with no progress.

Finally the senior midwife spoke to the junior doctor who decided to do a vacuum delivery and an episiotomy.

For Tara the negative 'birth territory' during labour and birth was experienced as a painful ordeal. The outcome for her was a very unhappy postnatal period with major postnatal depression. Tara did not breastfeed and did not bond well with the baby.

Interpretation of Tara's birth story

The description of Tara's birth encompasses much of what we know is important about environment. There was *no boundary* which the woman could *control*; *strangers* entered her space without her permission. There was *cold, hard furniture* which is neither inviting or nor comforting. The *bed and surgical light* created the sense of being a patient and needing to *submit to being dependent.* The *high technology medical equipment* probably created *fear.* The colours of the room, the artificial light and cool air temperature were outside Tara's control. We can assume that Tara's passive dependency is partly related to the unsupportive environment and her sense of *lack of control.* The lapse into sullen passivity certainly followed directly from *the midwives' refusal* to allow her epidural to be topped up and *the doctor's criticism* of her. This *loss of energy* and sense of victimhood is related to the uterus not contracting properly. This passive dependency is the antithesis of what birth requires of a woman; strength, courage and endurance. It is clear that Tara felt that she had no control over her environment and very little over her birth experience and that from the time she 'gave up' she had no chance of having a normal birth.

I acknowledge that this negative birth territory cannot, in a simple, reductionistic 'single-cause' way be 'blamed' for the negative outcomes for mother and baby. I am claiming that these experiences contributed to her sense of victimhood and depression and that this prevented her uterus from contracting properly and reduced her interest in and energy for birthing. I am claiming that a different birth experience may have had a healing effect on some of the past trauma and may have allowed her to avoid postnatal depression with the consequent lack of energy for early mothering.

LAPIS, A PRIMATE; BIRTHS IN A NATURAL ENVIRONMENT

Animals intuitively know that labour is a time of vulnerability to attack and so usually hide themselves away (Nisbett and Glander 1996). However, one fairly recent description of a free ranging primate, giving birth has been reported in the scientific literature. Observing a free ranging monkey giving birth in the natural environment is rare because birth normally takes place away from prying eyes and recording equipment. Up until 1988 there were no detailed published accounts but, in 1996, two biologists, who had been studying a group of Howler Monkeys for 20 years, finally observed and recorded the following birth (Nisbett and Glander 1996). They named the mother, Lapis. I have reproduced the original words of the researchers but have edited the description to eliminate unnecessary words; this is shown by tow square brackets, thus: [ ]. I also chose to simplify biological language and where I have done this I have put the synonym in **bold**.

Lapis: A Howler Monkey's story

At 13:50, Lapis walked into view **on all fours with her chest low,** her hind limbs wide **apart** and her back arched. She shuffled across the bough of a tree which the group used to cross a channel to a small island in **the river.** The rest of the group was already on the island but Lapis remained isolated on the crossing bough. [ ].

At 14:37 she raised her hands above her head and clinched her fists. She was restless, walking as described above [ ]. Five minutes later, using both hands she rubbed and pulled her vulva aggressively. She walked again, arching her **back** convexly. Two minutes later [ ], she contorted her **back** convexly, then concavely, grabbed her head and slapped her back with her tail, and finally wrapped her tail around her torso. Her abdomen was distended and she constantly moved and writhed.

At 14:45 she stood on all fours, unable to sit still, and then she sat in a hunched position. Two minutes later she climbed **another branch** holding her tail in hand. She shuffled along an oblique bough and then sat, clinching her fists.

At 14:48 she defecated and urinated; her vulva was very extended (added note, signs of second stage meaning that birth is near). Five minutes later she moved **on all fours** back out over the channel, pulling at her genitalia as she walked.

[ ] At 14:57 Lapis rose to an erect [ ] stand grasping the vines overhead. One minute later she returned to **an all fours** and arched her back again.

At 14:59 her vulva contracted, she walked to-and-fro, arching her back, and then sat. The whole anogenital region was protruding [ ]. At 15:00 she clenched her fists, manually inspected the vulva and then rose to an **all fours position.** She sat down one-half minutes later and rubbed her anogenital area with both hands.

At 15:00:45 she walked **on all fours,** sat, walked, sat [ ]. At 15:02, [ ] she **supported herself on all fours** and the head of the infant was partially visible. [ ]

At 15:05 she inspected her vulva **with her hands,** rubbing aggressively. She could not sit and leaned her left side against the **bough of the tree.** [ ] At 15:06:30 she rose from the leaning position onto **all fours** and, with abdominal contraction, much more of the infant's head became visible. [ ]. She tried to sit but could not and at 15:07 [ ] part of the infant's head emerged. [ ] Thirty seconds passed during which she continued to move during abdominal contraction.

At 15:08:30 the infant was expelled; amniotic fluids fell to the river below. The infant crawled onto her **front** generally unassisted although Lapis did cup it with her hands. [ ] One-half a minute later she moved across the limb toward an island in the river and became still for the first time in more than 30 minutes. The infant was cuddled on the **front.** She licked its face. **Three minutes later she was observed on the island with the tribe eating the placenta and cord. The rest of the group came to inspect the new baby.** Obvious labour and birth has taken a little over one and a quarter hours.

Interpretation of Lapis' birth in a natural environment

This description encompasses, some of what we know is important about 'birth territory'. To articulate just a few points; the *environment is natural* with no disruption of what the monkey usually experiences in day-to-day life, thus *culture is protected;* presumably this is *comforting or at least not frightening.* Lapis *created a boundary for herself by staying on the log but *her tribe was nearby.* Unlike Tara, she was allowed to have the jurisdiction over the area in which she birthed; *no one intruded.* Unlike Tara, *she was the one with the power* and she birthed independently. Note, *nothing happened to create fear or passivity* and

she felt free to move and behave exactly as her body prompted her to. This is critical to optimal physiological birthing. Consider how Lapis would feel and respond if someone came along and moved her to a clean, sterile, surgical environment? How might she feel if she was removed from her tribe and placed in a tribe of strangers for labour? If this happened I anticipate that, just as commonly happens for women experiencing medicalized birth, Lapis' contractions would have weakened and become incoordinate. Once that happened then her labour progress would be slow, the baby would become stressed inside the uterus and she would need medical attention to birth a live baby.

Some may argue that it is not appropriate to draw inferences about human physiology from other animals. Reproductive processes, however, involve the mammalian brain which, in humans, is the lower part of the brain and we share that part with all other mammals (Hardy 2000). In humans our innate, instinctive birthing behaviours, are over-ridden by our thinking, problem-solving brain. I am arguing that in labour the woman needs to let go of her thinking higher brain and respond moment to moment from her primitive mammalian brain. Dennis Walsh's research on nesting behaviours of women in birth centres add support to this notion (Walsh 2006b).

BARBARA'S BIRTH IN A HOME BIRTH ENVIRONMENT

The following description provided by Jenny Parratt, who was the woman's midwife, captures a home birthing environment that did work well for the woman. This is an extract from Jenny's journal (Parratt 2001):

Interpretation of Barbara's birth at home

This description encompasses some of what we know is important about the birth territory for humans and the woman's behaviour is remarkably similar to Lapis, described above. In this story the birthing woman owns the house where she is going to birth thus she *controls the boundaries* and who enters and leaves. Presumably she *felt safe, loved and supported. Her partner and the midwife can enforce* the woman's wishes when she is unable to do that for herself in late labour. As for the monkey the *environment is known*, it is non-clinical and presumably *comforting*; the woman's *chosen support people* were nearby but did *not interfere*, thus she felt *empowered* to birth independently; *nothing happened to create fea*r and she *felt free to move* and *behave exactly as she wished*. After birth she and the baby were *loved and welcomed by the family*. When Jenny checked a year later Barbara was happily breastfeeding. In spite of her previous history of depression, this time she experienced positive mental health in the postnatal period.

Barbara's story

Barbara lived in a new house on a small farm not far from a provincial city. She planned for her partner and their two-year-old daughter Shelly to be with her in labour. Barbara has had bouts of depression throughout her adult life. She felt physically and emotionally traumatized by her daughter's medicalized birth two years before this pregnancy. She experienced postnatal depression after her first child and antenatal depression during this pregnancy.

When the contractions started Barbara was preparing breakfast for Shelly. Throughout the day Barbara got on with her life moving from the kitchen, bedroom, bathroom, dressing her daughter and reading her a story. With each contraction she paused until the pain was gone. As the pain built and Barbara moved into the shower, where she began rocking and began to make noises. When I arrived she was on the mattress in the sitting room, on hands and knees with cushions around her. The fire was blazing and gentle winter sunlight filtered through the windows. Outside the dogs 'hovered' expectantly against the backdrop of a peaceful garden and sheep on the hills. Inside it was busy as Shelly and her Dad helped me unload equipment and call the other midwife.

Barbara was naked; she buried her head in the couch as each contraction rushed in on her. She began pushing with all her might. The second midwife quietly arrived. As the baby's head emerged from her body Barbara bent her head down so she could look between her legs to watch the birth of her baby. Barbara reached between her legs and caught him with the next contraction. I grabbed a towel to help her dry him off. Shelly and her dad were amazed and the four of them cuddled up close.

Barbara's baby was a healthy boy. She experienced no physical complications. She breastfed him and gave birth naturally to her placenta 50 minutes later.

Addendum, written in 2003: Barbara says she feels empowered. She is studying at university, has not had any depressive episodes and is still breastfeeding her son.

A BEGINNING THEORY OF BIRTH TERRITORY

'Birth territory' is comprised of a physical terrain of the birth space over which jurisdiction or power is claimed for the woman. The terrain denotes the physical, geographical and dynamic features of the individual birth space impacting on women and babies. Jurisdiction refers to power and how it is used in the birth space and beyond, including the way maternity services are organized and managed. Birth territories affect how women feel and respond as embodied beings; either they feel safe and loved or fearful and self-protective. The aim for the midwife is to skilfully create optimal environments within which women feel safe and where normal labour and birth physiology remain undisturbed.

In particular, birth territory refers to the features of the birth room, here termed the 'terrain', and the use of power within the room, here termed 'jurisdiction'.

Terrain

'Terrain' is a major sub-concept of birth territory. It denotes the physical features and geographical area of the individual birth space, including the furniture and fittings that the woman and her attendants use for labour and birth. Two sub-concepts, '**surveillance room**' and '**sanctum**', lie at opposite ends along this continuum called 'terrain'.

Sanctum
'**Sanctum**' is defined as a homely environment designed to optimize the privacy, ease and comfort of the woman; there is easy access to a toilet, a deep bath and access to or a view of the outdoors. Provision of a door that can close and lock from the inside meets the woman's need for privacy and safety. The more comfortable and familiar the environment is for the woman, the safer and more confident she will feel. An experience of 'sanctum' protects and potentially enhances the woman's embodied sense of self; this is reflected in optimal physiological function and emotional wellbeing.

Surveillance room
'**Surveillance room**' is the other sub-concept of 'terrain'. It denotes a clinical environment designed to facilitate surveillance of the woman and to optimize the ease and comfort of the staff. This is relevant to the concept of 'jurisdiction' (discussed below) and it is consistent with Foucault's notion of disciplinary power. A 'surveillance room' is a clinical-looking room where equipment the staff may need is on display and the bed dominates. It has a doorway but no closed door, or the door has a viewing window so the staff can see into the room (not so the woman can look out). The woman has no easy access to bath, toilet or the outdoors.

Proposition

The more a birth room deviates from a 'sanctum', the more likely it is that the woman will feel fear. This deviation from the 'sanctum' will in turn reduce her sense of self it will be reflected in inhibited physiological functioning, reduced emotional wellbeing and possibly emotional distress.

Jurisdiction

'Jurisdiction' means having the power to do as one wants within the birth environment. 'Power' is an energy which enables one to be able to do or obtain what one wants (Northrup 1998). Power is essential for living; without it we would not move at all. Power is ethically neutral; this is consistent with Foucault's notion of power which he argued was productive; not necessarily oppressive (Foucault 1980). Power can be used to get others to submit to one's own wishes. Health professionals who want women to submit to their authority (to be docile) normally use a subtle form of coercive power that Foucault called 'disciplinary power'. The concept of jurisdiction is directly relevant to 'midwifery guardianship' which is the topic of the next chapter in which the theory of birth territory continues to be developed.

CONCLUSIONS

Unlike Lapis, most women live in houses and do not fully retreat to birth. Indeed most contemporary women want to know how they and their babies are progressing in labour. Further, women want to know that if they need medical assistance in birth that they can obtain it easily. The important point is that in spite of wanting the benefits of obstetrics when needed women do not want to be put under surveillance and taken over by obstetric rules and procedures. There is a real difference between having your baby 'delivered' and 'giving birth'. Having your baby delivered induces feelings of dependency, weakness and gratitude to others while giving birth promotes feelings of love, strength and self-confidence. There is a middle path for modern women; to create a birth sanctum. A sanctum can be created in either a birth centre or a home that is near to a maternity hospital. In these birth settings midwives provide relatively unobtrusive monitoring of woman who are giving birth and they can refer quickly and easily to medicine if required.

The next chapter will focus on the role of the midwife in protecting and supporting women to access and use their inner power to birth instinctively.

QUESTIONS FOR DISCUSSION

1. Do you think the comparison of a monkey's birth to a woman's birth is justified? Why/why not?

2. How important is it, in your view, that the woman, or her midwife, can control who enters and leaves the room? Why/why not?

3. The author of this chapter implicated the birth territory for Tara's birth in her subsequent postnatal depression. Do you think that is justified? Why/why not?

4. How important is it that the woman knows and trusts the people in the birthing room? Why/why not?
   This is better covered by the more positive frame up of the next question – you don't want them to focus on what they don't need, but what they do need.

5. Considering your local maternity unit, to what extent do the birth rooms reflect the characteristics of a sanctum for birth?

References

Cunningham G 2005 William's obstetrics. New York, McGraw-Hill.

Fahy K 1995 Marginalised mothers: Teenage transition to motherhood and the experience of disciplinary power. Anthropology and Sociology. University of Queensland, Brisbane, p. 395.

Fahy K, Parratt J 2006 Birth territory: a theory for midwifery practice. Women and Birth 19(2): 45–50.

Foucault M 1980 Power/knowledge: selected interviews. Pantheon, New York.

Friedan B 1963 The feminine mystique. W.W. Norton, New York.

Gould D 2002 Birthwrite: Subliminal medicalisation. British Journal of Midwifery 10(7): 418.

Grosz E 1994 Volatile bodies: Towards a corporeal feminism. Indiana University Press, Bloomington.

Hardy S B 2000 Mother nature. Random House, London.

Irigaray L 1985 Speculum of the other woman. Translated by Gilligan C. Ithaca, New York.

Johnson P 1994 Feminism as radical humanism. Allen and Unwin, Sydney.

Kristeva J 1995 New maladies of the soul. Translated by Ross Guberman. Columbia University Press, New York.

Mellor A 2003 Feminist Theory. Encyclopedia of the enlightenment. Alan Charles Kors, Ed. Oxford University Press 2003. http://0-www.oxfordreference.com.library. newcastle.edu.au:80/views/ENTRY.html?subview= Main&entry=t173.e222 Accessed 10 October 2006.

NCT 2003 Improving the built environment and culture for birth. The National Childbirth Trust, London.

Nisbett R, Glander K 1996 Quantitative description of parturition in a wild mantled howling monkey: A case study of prenatal behaviors associated with primiparous delivery. Brenesia 45–46: 157–168.

Northrup C 1998 Women's bodies, women's wisdom. Bath, Piatkus.

Onions C 2002 Shorter Oxford English Dictionary, University Press, Oxford.

Parratt J 2001 Journal entry.

Stanley S, Wise L 1993 Breaking out again: Feminist ontology and epistemology. Routledge, London.

Walsh D 2000 Part five: Why we should reject the 'bed birth' myth. British Journal of Midwifery 8(9): 554–558.

Walsh D 2006a Subverting the assembly-line: Childbirth in a free-standing birth centre. Social Science and Medicine 62(6): 1330–1336.

Walsh D 2006b Nesting and matrescence as distinctive features of a free-standing birth centre in the UK. Midwifery 22(3): 228–239.

Whitford M, Ed. 1991 The Irigaray reader. Blackwell, Cambridge.

Wolf N 1993 Fire with fire: The new female power and how it will change the 21st century. Chatto & Windus, London.

Young I M 2005 On female body experience: Throwing like a girl and other essays. Oxford University Press, Oxford.

Chapter **3**

Midwifery guardianship: Reclaiming the sacred in birth

Kathleen Fahy
Carolyn Hastie

Across time and cultures, women's knowledge has included great wisdom about birth. That knowledge has been virtually lost in the Western world. In Western science only that which can be seen, weighed and counted is considered real. Any other sort of knowledge is discounted and excluded. Writing about the role of the midwife guardian, who creates and maintains spiritually and emotionally safe birth spaces, has felt like reclaiming something very valuable. This chapter gives words to the embodied wisdom of women and midwives and does so in a way that links that knowledge to other forms of scholarly and scientific knowledge.

A discussion of power as it relates to midwifery guardianship begins the chapter. Niki's birth story is then used to make explicit how power is operating within the woman and within the birth territory. The spiritual foundations for midwifery guardianship are next described and related to psycho-analytic concepts including ego and inner self. The importance of love and self-nurturing are explored in relation to midwifery guardians, promoting the integration of ego and inner self for themselves as well as for women. The importance of women experiencing non-ordinary consciousness states in birth is discussed and applied by the use of clinical examples. Finally, the ethical aspects of caring for women, particularly during non-ordinary states of consciousness are considered.

THE CONCEPT OF INTEGRATIVE POWER

'Integrative power' integrates all forms of power within the environment to some shared higher goal. The primary aim of using 'integrative power' is to support integration of the woman's body, mind and spirit so that she feels able to respond spontaneously and expressively to her bodily sensations and intuitions. The integration of mind–body–spirit increases her energy, strength and power.

When the woman needs to make decisions about her options during the birth process, the conscious use of 'integrative power' by all participants in the birth territory promotes the best birthing psychology, physiology and outcomes. In that state of integrated group consciousness, all power is focused on the woman's enhanced mind–body–spirit integration and consequently, on her self-expression and confidence in being the one who is making the ultimate choice about what happens. Importantly, the use of 'integrative power' supports the woman to feel good about her self even if the birth outcome is not as she had wished.

Midwifery guardianship

'Midwifery guardianship' is a sub-concept of 'integrative power' which allows midwives to exercise jurisdiction over the birth territory. Midwifery guardians are embodied selves (see Chapter 4) who access their various forms of power, including inner power to create and maintain harmony between themselves and the woman and within the birthing room. Midwifery guardianship involves controlling who crosses the boundaries of the birth space in line with the wishes of the woman. The desired outcome of midwifery guardianship is that women feel strong and empowered even if the birth is not as they had wished or planned.

A 'midwifery guardian' works with the woman to slow down her everyday thinking mind and focus mindfully on her baby, her body and the birthing process. In neurophysiological terms, this means assisting the woman to become relaxed and focused in a non-ordinary consciousness state which is discussed further below.

DISINTEGRATIVE POWER

'Disintegrative power' is an ego-centred power that disintegrates other forms of power within the environment and imposes the user's self-serving goal. It may be used by the woman, the midwife and/or any other person in the territory. When disintegrative power is used by the woman it is an ego-based determination to have a particular experience or outcome. Regardless of who uses it, disintegrative power undermines the woman's ability to be able to feel, trust and respond spontaneously to her bodily sensations and intuitions. This is a disintegration of the woman's mind–body–spirit unity that separates her from her embodied power thus weakening her and lowering her energy.

Niki's story

The story to follow demonstrates a relatively ideal 'birth territory'. In the story you are invited to focus on the powers in play in the situation and to see how Niki needs to be the one with the power. Real names have been used with permission. This story has been checked and validated by Niki, Carolyn and Andrew. The authors of this chapter were the midwives at this birth. The story has previously been published as part of a journal article (Fahy and Parratt 2006). Interpretive comments that link to the theoretical concepts of birth territory are *in italics*.

Niki was having her first baby. Labour had begun with the baby's head in an occipito-transverse position, this is

not unusual, many babies start labour in this position. We assumed the baby would rotate naturally according to the normal mechanism of labour. Niki used the deep birth pool for eight hours using meditation techniques to cope with the sensations of labour. Gavin (Niki's partner) was a quiet, loving and supportive presence. Carolyn (the other midwife) and I were quiet and unobtrusive; however, in line with medical protocols we recorded Niki's blood pressure second hourly and assessed her pulse and the baby's heart rate every 15 minutes. *The 'jurisdiction' of the space is Niki's and the midwives are acting as midwifery guardians.*

Niki's story   Continued

All went well until transition which continued for about 3 hours. During the first part of this time Niki wanted to get out of the bath and change positions and we encouraged her to follow this instinct. *'Integrative power' is being used by Niki and the midwives.*

As the time progressed and we saw no signs of second stage, Carolyn suggested that Niki move her hips in particular ways to assist with pelvic opening and optimal fetal positioning. With great strength, courage and endurance, Niki followed Carolyn's advice and squatted, lunged, walked, used hands and knees positions and the birth stool; all to no avail. *This is a use of integrative power; it brings midwifery power/knowledge to the situation and integrates with the power of the woman and her body.*

We discussed with Niki and Gavin that on palpation the baby's head was still in the deflexed occipito-transverse position. A vaginal examination confirmed that the head was deflexed and in the occipito-transverse position at the spines and may be caught up on the spines. As the cervix was not yet fully dilated, the obstetrician (Andrew), whom they knew a little, suggested to Niki that she may want to have an epidural and her contractions strengthened by the use of a Syntocinon infusion. *Andrew's use of power/ knowledge is integrative as it leaves the choice of having both the epidural and Syntocinon up to Niki.*

These words had an almost immediate effect on Niki. She turned on her side, went physically limp as if giving up, and cried. She said, 'I don't want Syntocinon'. Up until this point Niki had been strong and active, suddenly she appeared weak and passive. *Niki's ego-based determination to have a particular experience has created 'disintegrative power' that has undermined her embodied sense of self causing a loss of power illustrated by her weakened passivity.*

Carolyn spoke firmly to her. 'No, Niki, you don't have to have Syntocinon. There are midwifery strategies that we can try, you can still have a normal birth, but we need you to be here and fully present'. *This is a call to be mindful; to bring the mind and the body together in harmony.* 'You need to come back here right now and you need to be strong and courageous. I want you to get up and start moving'. 'Gavin', she directed, 'I want you to come and help Niki'. 'Andrew', she continued, and turned to him, 'can you give us 40 minutes please and come back then?' Andrew agreed and quietly left the room. *This is the midwife and obstetrician using integrative power.*

Carolyn moves to reverse Niki's use of disintegrative power; she uses integrative power to call for Niki's fully embodied presence.

The effect of Carolyn's powerful intervention was amazing. Niki regained her strength and confidence. With fortitude and grace Niki got up and started moving as Carolyn instructed. She began stepping sideways up the steps of the birth pool with Gavin providing physical and psychological support. After a time Carolyn advised squatting for a few contractions and Niki did this, again with Gavin's loving support. This movement went on for the next 40 minutes of labour with all of us actively involved in supporting Niki and listening to the baby's heart sounds every 15 minutes. *This is integrative power in action.*

During this time Niki's facial expressions showed she was in pain, but she didn't complain or cry out; she was too busy putting all her energy into helping her pelvis to open and the baby to turn. *This is evidence of her greater mind–body–spirit integration and enhanced embodied sense of self.*

After talking quietly together, Carolyn and I agreed that there were three options if the head did not rotate within the 40 minutes allocated. We discussed them with Niki and Gavin before Andrew returned. *This is integrative power because we were sharing our knowledge and predictions with Niki and Gavin in advance of when they would need the knowledge so that they could be prepared.*

When Andrew got back he examined Niki and found her fully dilated, but the head was still in the deflexed occipito-transverse position. At this point all five of us discussed the three options for moving forward. Niki chose a manual rotation. Andrew said it might be too painful but he was willing to try if Niki was. With Niki sitting on the birth stool Andrew performed a manual rotation when Niki had a contraction. The head moved easily into the correct position and baby Declan was born normally about two hours later. *This is the use of integrative power.*

Immediately after birth, Niki, Gavin and baby Declan were bonding beautifully; nearly two hours later Niki birthed the placenta physiologically with minimal blood loss and they went home after four hours. Niki and Gavin described amazing feelings of being overwhelmed with love for Declan. Niki was proud of herself and very pleased with Gavin's support in labour. Gavin was proud of Niki and himself; they were both thrilled with the outcome. Niki and Declan proceeded to have a positive postnatal and breastfeeding experience.

POWER AND BIRTH

Niki, Gavin and I discussed the birth about a week afterwards. They were convinced that the respectful and positive care that they received prevented a caesarean section. When asked how she felt about Carolyn's forceful intervention asking her to be strong, get moving and not give up, Niki said 'I thought she was great because she made me feel that what I wanted (a normal birth) was possible, that I didn't have to give up. Someone else who really knew about birth believed in me and in my dream and I was able to trust myself again and to keep on going'. *This was evidence of how midwifery guardianship and integrative power can harness the woman's own power while using midwifery and medical interventions only as they are specifically needed.*

Birth territory and midwifery guardianship weren't the only factors involved in creating the positive outcomes for Niki and her family. She had experienced continuity of carer with her midwives and knew us both well. In addition, she had personal characteristics that were central to her outcomes: she was middle class, university educated, a qualified yoga instructor and regular yoga practitioner, in a happy and supportive partnership; had read widely; had discussed birthing options fully with her midwives; was open to ideas and she was committed to natural birth. The story above and Niki's own words demonstrate however, that Niki would have been most unlikely to have given birth normally had she been cared for in a 'surveillance room' without midwifery guardianship.

THE SPIRITUAL FOUNDATIONS OF MIDWIFERY GUARDIANSHIP

Some of the ideas in this section on 'spirituality', 'universal energy' and the 'inner self' are not referenced in the usual scholarly way. That is because most of the ideas that are presented here have been synthesized over many years of practising, reading, meditating, praying, living and reflecting. We have engaged in long conversations with each other and with other spiritual seekers. Even though the ideas are difficult to articulate and open to both criticism and individual interpretation, we offer our current understandings. We believe our conception of spirituality is broadly consistent with interpretations of quantum physics, Jung's (1960) and Grof's (1985) psychoanalytical psychology, some non-fundamentalist forms of Christianity, as well as Eastern Philosophy and Spirituality, including Hinduism, Buddhism and Taoism.

Spirituality

Humans long to feel whole or connected with the sacred dimensions of life. Sometimes this quest is towards something bigger and more powerful than us and sometimes the quest is inwards, towards knowing our inner self more fully. The quest for wholeness and connection is termed 'spirituality'. Spiritual experience refers to our direct, personal encounters with universal energy and the sacred dimension of existence. A peak spiritual experience sometimes occurs during birth. A peak spiritual experience is one in which one ecstatically transcends the usual limited perspective of self and life (Maslow 1964; Grof 1985, 1993; Taylor 1995; Kornfield 2002). From a spiritual perspective, universal energy is the animating energy that drives all activity within the universe. Universal energy is part of all living and non-living things. This energy is expanding and is everywhere; it is all that is or ever was. Universal energy is ethically neutral although humans often seek to label it good and evil depending upon how we value the material expression of universal energy (Jung 1960; Maslow 1964; Grof 1985, 1993; Taylor 1995; Khor 2004).

The characteristics of ego

The concepts of 'ego' and 'inner self' are a necessary part of understanding the transformative power and spirituality of birth (see Chapter 4 for more details).

Ego is a construct that was developed by Freud and continues to be a mainstay concept for psychoanalytic psychology and psychiatry. Psychoanalytic theories investigate and explain the interaction of conscious and unconscious elements in the mind. Psychoanalytic practice includes bringing repressed fears and conflicts into the conscious mind so that the emotional charge associated with them can be reframed and released (Moore 2004).

In the section that follows we concentrate on the characteristics of ego, but it is important to know that there is no pure state of ego without inner self or vice versa. Ego is a vital part of self but can cause us problems if it becomes so dominant that the softer inner self can't make itself known.

Ego is that part of the self which is made up of a set of roles and identities which were developed in response to the self's embodied socialization. Ego is bounded by time, space and the five senses. Ego looks outwards to other people or things to find meaning, learning, happiness and help. Ego is rational and conceptual; frequently considering the past and the future at the expense of the present time. Ego breaks everything down into dichotomies: e.g. right vs. wrong, win vs. lose and strong vs. weak. Ego wants answers to questions like 'why', 'how much', 'how many' and 'how long'?

Ego thinks a lot about the past and worries a lot about the future. In an attempt to feel peaceful and satisfied, ego grasps at and clings to people and things outside itself, leading to addiction and unhealthy attachments. Ego tries to predict what the other/s want from us and then to work out the safest course of action in order to avoid being hurt, humiliated or abandoned.

Ego is ethically neutral; we need ego in order to play out our social roles and duties. Ego knows the rules; it knows how to play the games that our cultures require. In some life situations, it is in our best interests that ego is dominant; for example when operating machinery or needing to work within the law. In other situations it is in our higher best interest if ego is quiet and the inner self is able to take the lead. The inner self should lead, for example when we are: feeling and expressing love and sexuality; giving birth; healing from illness and dying. Ego can only interfere at times like these. We would find that instead of being authentic and true to our inner self, if ego was dominant then we would act out roles and look to others to see how we are going from their point of view.

Ego can be thought of as a set of stimulus–response tapes where the 'play' button is pressed each time ego is activated by some external stimulus. What we are calling stimulus–response tapes are actually biological patterns of neural activity involving the whole body. Learning and associated emotions are encoded in these patterns of neural activity (Berry Brazelton 1983; Winnicot 1988; Mauger 1998; Siegal 1999; Schore 2002; Lipton 2005). Each neural network pattern is specific to a particular environmental stimulus and when that stimulus, or something similar presents, the neural network fires, releasing messenger molecules, creating an emotional state that motivates an ego response. These egoic patterned ways of responding were developed in childhood and are used in adult life mostly unconsciously.

For example, if a child is being abused by her parent, it is helpful for her to be docile and submissive and to believe that her parent still loves her. The belief is important, even life-saving because a loving child is more likely to be cared for and survive than an angry or aggressive child. The belief is an 'ego defence mechanism'. 'Ego defence mechanisms are coping styles that are employed automatically and most often unconsciously to protect the individual from becoming aware of internal and external dangers or anxieties' (Taylor 1995, p. 236). When the child in this scenario grows up she is likely to find herself in relationships that mirror her childhood experience, for example domestic violence. And, without some psycho-spiritual development she will employ the same ego defence mechanism that worked for her in childhood to keep her safe and alive. Now, as an adult, however, she can choose to look after her own survival needs. As this scenario shows, ego's reasoning can often be faulty, because its version of reality is perceived through defence mechanisms of its own making. These defence mechanisms, such as idealizing, fantasizing, judging, blaming or rationalizing, protect ego from facing reality because ego thinks (wrongly) that reality is too frightening or too shaming (Jung 1960; Grof 1985; Taylor 1995; Kornfield 2002).

Egoic power

Whenever ego detects that the environment is less than totally safe, ego may seek to hide any sign of vulnerability and use 'egoic power'. Using egoic power may mean exerting control over other people, over one's inner self and/or over one's own body. The unfettered use of egoic power is dominating, defensive and/or combative. Exercising 'egoic power' involves grasping at or holding on to what one's ego has or wants.

Egoic power is narrowly fixed on a particular goal without consciousness of the possible negative consequences of getting what ego wants. When a person is operating from their egoic power, it expresses itself by using energy that is 'hard', 'determined' or 'manipulative' of others in order to get what he/she wants and to block out other knowledge or possibilities. Power from ego is often about winning or proving a point to oneself or someone else. When women hold on to egoic control in childbirth it means that they miss out on the empowering spiritual transformation that is possible only when it involves the woman fully; i.e. mind–body–spirit. Two fictionalized examples show ego's narrow focus and use of disintegrative, egoic power, to get a particular outcome. It is disintegrative because it cut the woman off from her inner self and from other sources of knowledge and wisdom.

Daphne's story

Daphne had never experienced herself as strong or competent. As a child she got what she wanted by appearing weak, needy and dependent. Her parents felt sorry for her and helped her so she would feel better. Not surprisingly when she began labouring in her first birth, her usual egoic way of coping asserted herself. Before labour was even well-established she was lying down on the bed moaning and crying.
'I can't cope with this,' she lamented. Daphne begged the midwives to help her. The midwives encouraged Daphne to feel strong, to get upright, to start moving, to use the bath, but Daphne then began to say, in a 'baby-like' voice, that it was all too hard, that she wanted an epidural. The midwives told her an epidural would likely stop the labour; that an oxytocin drip and possibly a caesarean would be the end result, but Daphne begged them to help her. She got her epidural and also the oxytocin and continuous fetal monitoring. The baby needed medical assistance to be born because Daphne couldn't feel to push and felt too tired. The baby needed to be resuscitated and spent a day in the nursery. Breastfeeding didn't go well; it was all too hard for Daphne. Later she developed postnatal depression.

Gemma's story

Gemma was so determined to avoid losing control that she chose a caesarean birth without a medical indication. She used her ego to block out consciousness regarding what the obstetrician said about the possibility that the baby may develop respiratory distress because of a caesarean birth. Equally, she ignored the possibility that she may get any of the serious postoperative complications that he told her about. Following the elective caesarean the baby had to be admitted to intensive care with lung complications. Gemma developed a wound infection that resulted in a complete breakdown of her wound a week after birth. When she became pregnant for a second time, the placenta grew into the old caesarean scar. This caused bleeding in pregnancy that resulted in an emergency caesarean at 27 weeks gestation. Gemma needed multiple blood transfusions and a hysterectomy to correct her shock and blood loss. The premature baby needed many weeks of intensive care nursery.

Table 3.1 will assist you to be able to discern which form of power is leading in childbirth: egoic or inner power.

Characteristics of the inner self

The 'inner self' is the 'spirit', that energetic, electromagnetic part of self which existed prior to conception and which is part of universal energy. Like universal energy the inner self is ethically neutral. The inner self is non-verbal, non-rational, creative, timeless, limitless, intuitive, wise and powerful. The inner self accesses feelings to express itself, communicates symbolically (Maslow 1964; Grof 1985, 1993; Taylor 1995). The inner self expresses itself through the body in sound and movement and symbolically or metaphorically; for example in art, visions and dreams. The inner self sends subtle signals which we experience as bodily feelings. Sensing and responding to these feelings we are able to know how to respond in ways that are most healthful and resourceful.

Inner power
'Inner power' is 'integrative' of mind–body–spirit and respectful of the mind–bodies of all other people. Inner power prompts the self towards

Table 3.1 Discerning the chief source of power in birthing

Signs that ego is in charge during birthing	Signs that the inner self is leading during birthing
The woman: • is alert or hyper alert • is talkative • is orientated in time and place • worries about how she will cope in the future • judges self and others • thinks about how others perceive her • attempts to be in control • thinks about people or things outside self • attempts to be rational and avoid emotionality • feels powerful or powerless • feels tired or worries about feeling tired • forces things to happen (or attempts to) • assumes the positions and behaviours that are expected • experiences labour contractions as pain and suffering • wants to cut off from or stop the pain and/or just wants it all over • complains about the experience • if she verbalizes, is seeking sympathy	The woman: • is dreamily defenceless • is silent or noisy; not 'chatty' • is largely unaware of time and place • deals with each moment as it arises • is non-judgmental • is unconcerned about how others perceive her • has surrendered control to her body and the environment • focuses inward and senses bodily feelings without judging or trying to control them • lets go of rationality and embraces emotionality • feels she has enough power • feels she has enough energy • allows labour to progress at its own rate and in its own way • moves and expresses intuitively to bodily signals • may experience contractions as power surges rather than pain • welcomes each contraction and sensation as one step closer to holding her baby • focuses on the experience without complaint • if she verbalizes, does so in an honest way of expressing her experience, says 'it hurts!' or 'ow' as a releasing mechanism

more of everything that life has to offer. The mind is required to trust the process enough to allow the whole self, mind–body–spirit to go with the energy (flow). The power of the inner self can only be accessed by surrendering egoic attempts to control. Inner power is accessed rather than exercised. Inner power is an energy that moves the self to take action which is sensed to be in the higher interests of the whole self and sometimes also others. Taking action towards one's own or another's best interests is acting from 'love'.

Love   Love is an expression of universal energy, the inner self and inner power. When we 'love' it is experienced as a feeling of open-heartedness which the Buddhists call loving-compassion (Kornfield 2002). Our understanding of love is similar in some respects to M. Scott Peck's definition and we agree with him that love is expressed through extending one's self for the purpose of nurturing one's own or another's psycho-spiritual growth (Peck 1993). Love may include the expression of affection by words, symbols or actions. Love needs to be discriminated from other motives that masquerade as love because

they cause us to be confused about how someone is feeling towards us, e.g. clinging, dependence, fear, control and jealousy are not love. When these emotions are motivating the supposed loving behaviour, the effect on the beloved may be discerned by that person experiencing personal stagnation or disintegration (Peck 1993; Goleman 2003). Consider, for example, an abusive partner or an overly controlling parent.

Love isn't just about psycho-spiritual growth but also includes biological growth and wellbeing. Thus love is operating where the one doing the loving is promoting the health, happiness, wellbeing and consciousness of the beloved. Loving in the manner we mean it, is a process of extending oneself, which, when the love is accepted, results in both the lover and the beloved growing as a consequence. Women need to be loved and supported by a midwife. The relationship is a form of professional friendship that begins and ends with childbearing. In order for midwives to be able to form healthy and loving relationship with many women over their professional careers they need to ensure that their own needs are met. All forms of loving begin with and emanate from self-love.

Accessing the inner self via non-ordinary consciousness

Experiencing non-ordinary states of consciousness in birth is common because women experience these states spontaneously; particularly if the midwife feels confident of supporting women in those states (Paul and Paul 1975; Green et al 1990; Lahood 2007). (See Chapter 4 for more details.)

Non-ordinary states of consciousness can be considered in two broad categories; 'delirium' and 'holotrophic'. Delirium is an organic disorder precipitated by brain disease, fever, metabolic disorder or drugs or alcohol intoxication. Delirium is characterized as 'an acutely disordered state of mind involving incoherent speech, hallucinations, and frenzied excitement' (Moore 2004). In comparison, holotrophic non-ordinary states of consciousness may share some or all of the observable characteristics of delirium, but they are temporary and there is no underlying precipitating disease state or intoxication. During a holotrophic state of non-ordinary consciousness the person experiences a process of re-organizing attitudes, values, beliefs and behaviours in a way that moves towards healing and wholeness. During the process of re-organizing, it may seem as though the mind is disordered in relation to everyday consensual reality, but this is a temporary and healthful state (Grof 1985).

Holotrophic non-ordinary states of consciousness occur regularly and spontaneously throughout life, e.g. dreaming, performing some activity you love where time and place are lost such as painting, writing, sculpting, meditating or having an orgasm. Pregnancy, in most cultures, is a ritual state which is treated as sacred and is accompanied by specific rites (Kitzinger 1978). These rites are thought to assist pregnant women to access the altered states necessary to birth well. Bourguignon (1973) an anthropologist, found that 90% of cultures have institutionalized rituals to assist people to enter deeper non-ordinary or trance states. Indigenous cultures from around the world continue to have socially sanctioned ways for people to 'reverently and regularly enter non-ordinary states of consciousness' (Taylor 1994; Lahood 2007).

Recognizing non-ordinary states of consciousness

Table 3.2 provides the defining characteristics of ordinary, mild non-ordinary and deep non-ordinary states of consciousness (Taylor 1995) which we will be referring to throughout the rest of this chapter. It is important to realize that these states are not fixed or rigid; people typically move between the various levels of consciousness.

Responding to spiritual emergence in birth All humans have the potential to grow and develop throughout their lives but birth, particularly first birth, is a powerful time of spiritual emergence for women. In transpersonal psychology (Grof and Grof 1989) the term 'process' is used to describe psycho-spiritual insights, emotions, changes, methods and integration towards increasing consciousness. Most women experience the

Table 3.2   Recognizing non-ordinary states of consciousness (based on Taylor, 1994)

Ordinary state	Mild non-ordinary	Deep non-ordinary
Alert	Is in reverie	Has difficulty functioning in an ordinary way
Talks easily	Able to speak if needed	May have difficulty speaking
In touch with consensual reality	Not thinking about consensual reality unless asked	Has less ability to express experiences in words
Eyes open	Eyes usually closed	Eyes closed
Clear sense of time	Time may be lost	Time distortion
Clear sense of self and others	Sense of self may blur	Self may be experienced at a different time in biography or in the transpersonal realm
Aware of surroundings	May lose sense of surroundings	Has less reference points for ordinary reality
	Can relatively quickly re-focus and switch to ordinary consciousness	Has access to deeper levels of healing
		Has access to mystical states

childbearing year as a time of rapid growth and development; this is particularly true of undisturbed labour and birth where non-ordinary states of consciousness occur. When a person enters non-ordinary consciousness their 'process' is likely to intensify and they may experience a number of different states on the way to 'spiritual emergence'. A spiritual emergence is the psycho-spiritual development of the self, involving major changes in beliefs, emotions, insight and relationship to body, others, the world and God (Taylor 1995). Spiritual emergence is a process that is accompanied by increased wisdom, power and insight. Spiritual emergence is a beneficial state that may not be achieved without experiencing less positive states along the path. Some of these states are mentioned here.

A 'spiritual emergency', in contrast, involves rapid and dramatic psycho-spiritual development in which the person becomes partially or fully dysfunctional for a period of time (Grof and Grof 1989; Taylor 1995). Spiritual emergency may present in labour as 'dissociation' which is sometimes called 'splitting'. Dissociation is an ego defence to protect the self from physical or emotional overwhelm. Dissociation is internal disconnection between thoughts and feelings or intuitions or sensations or between one part of self and another (Taylor 1995). 'Severe dissociation may involve multiplicity, which is the psychic state where parts of the personality and memory are separated from other parts' (Taylor 1995). Women who have been sexually abused may experience this type of dissociation in labour (Parratt 1993).

When dissociation happens during labour it may present as trauma re-enactment (Parratt 1993). Trauma re-enactment involves 'reliving the same pattern of trauma experienced earlier in life' (Taylor 1995). Childbirth has the potential for healing past traumas that arise spontaneously. The conditions for healing are a safe setting and experienced, sensitive, professional midwifery support. Additionally the client needs to be aware that what is occurring is a trauma re-enactment based on neural network activation from implicit memory triggered by the physical experience of labour and birth. If, however, trauma re-enactment arises but the woman remains unconscious to its meaning, it can be

damaging to her as she experiences it as a repeat victimization. Some women actually experience additional victimization in labour and birth when unwanted or painful procedures are performed upon them, e.g. vaginal examination, forceps delivery or being held down or restrained in any way.

An important idea for both women and midwives to have is 'witness consciousness' which is a part of self that can serve our highest good by observing and mediating between ego and inner self. Our witness normally continues to operate even when we are in non-ordinary states of consciousness. During non-ordinary consciousness our witness gives us permission to let go of ego control. Our witness continues to watch us as we feel and behave differently from what we do in ordinary consciousness. If our witness detects that the situation we are in is less than fully safe for mind–body–spirit, then the witness marshals the full force of ego to come to our protection and defence (Grof 1985; Taylor 1994). Thus, in labour, if a woman is in a non-ordinary state when her witness detects that a person in her birth territory is unsafe physically or emotionally, then she may snap out of her non-ordinary state in order to have her ego defend her safety. If a woman experiences dissociation, the midwife needs to speak calmly and warmly to that part of the woman which is her 'witness consciousness'.

Example of a holotrophic non-ordinary state in birth

Lennie's story

Lennie desperately wanted to avoid intervention in labour and birth. This was her first baby. Lennie had many hours of inner struggle. She had been willing her body to relax and give birth while simultaneously engaging in trying to control the process. This had the effect of labour stopping and starting; the all too familiar (to me) 'failure to progress' scenario which happens when women are internally divided against themselves. Finally Lennie succumbed to an epidural and Syntocinon. Even with the epidural, she remained stalled in labour and facing a caesarean if she didn't show signs of progress in the next hour. I suggested that she may like to accept that possibility rather than resisting it. I suggested that she work on talking to the baby and imagining the baby being born normally.

Lennie's story   Continued

Lennie cried and finally surrendered to the possibility of a caesarean simultaneously letting go of ego control. She closed her eyes and focused on breathing slowly and deeply. She told me later that she 'went somewhere I have never been before' inside herself, somewhere 'very peaceful' (i.e. a non-ordinary state of consciousness). When Lennie was examined an hour later, she was fully dilated and the baby was ready to be born. Lennie went on to birth her baby and placenta beautifully, with her perineum intact. Breathing slowly and deeply is one of the ways you can significantly reduce your stress reaction and engage your relaxation response with state associated positive neuro-hormonal and muscular effects.

Differentiating the ego from the inner self

Being able to discern the difference between whether the ego or the inner self is leading the woman in labour is part of what a midwife and woman need to know in order to birth safely. When a woman is in a non-ordinary state of consciousness and in touch with her inner power and subconscious processes, the midwife needs to be in an ordinary state of consciousness so that she is able to discern the source and potential effect of the expression of the 'inner power'. The importance of the midwife remaining centred and in a normal state of consciousness is discussed in the following section about being able to discern what is happening during the woman's non-ordinary states.

Ego getting in the way of birth

Rachel's story

Rachel was in labour with her second baby; she had her husband, Tim and both sets of parents with her. Labour wasn't progressing and in discussion with her midwife (Carolyn), Rachel recognized her inability to 'let go' with everyone present. She said she just couldn't ask them to leave (no doubt because she feared the long-term consequences of hurting their feelings). I (Carolyn) encouraged the parents to leave and explained the hormonal cascade and the need for most women to feel unobserved for labour to progress. The parents didn't believe me and refused to leave. Tim, Rachel's husband felt powerless to contradict the families. Eventually Rachel's

contractions 'fizzled out' and she went home two hours later. The next evening, Rachel came into the birth suite with only Tim accompanying her. This time she could relax and let go and progressed rapidly to give birth three hours later. Rachel and Tim didn't ring the families until the baby was six hours old. Rachel said it took two months for them all to forgive her and for relationships to get back to normal.

Kelly's story

Kelly, on the other hand, wanted everyone to be present for the birth of her baby. Every time a labour surge occurred, Kelly would look around at everyone to ensure they were all looking at her (egoic control). She demanded back rubs, hot packs, water etc constantly. Kelly and her support team acted like it was one big party. There was no space for Kelly to enter the deep focused internal state of mind needed to access her 'inner self' and 'inner power'. Her partner couldn't bear seeing Kelly in pain and begged her to have an epidural. She agreed, pleased with all the attention she was getting. Kelly's cervical dilatation was slow even after medical attempts to stimulate with rupturing membranes and using an oxytocic intravenously. Kelly was told that she would require a caesarean if she wasn't fully dilated at the next examination in one hour's time. As Kelly went off to the operating theatre an hour later she was crying because all her support people were going to miss the birth (again showing her external egoic focus).

Sylvia's story

Sylvia was rocking her hips back and forward, leaning over a chair. She was groaning through her contractions. Sylvia was having her fourth baby and was expressing some impatience that birth wasn't happening 'quickly enough' (ego dominance). I (Carolyn) asked her what she was saying to herself. She told me she was saying 'baby's coming, welcome baby!' (could be inner-self but might be Sylvia giving me the 'right' answer). I noted she didn't look me in the eye when she said that, so I suspected that this wasn't the whole truth. From experience I suspected that Sylvia had another internal conversation going on. I asked her what was the other part of herself saying? Sylvia looked at me like a naughty child who had been 'caught out'. She laughed and said 'it's

Sylvia's story   Continued

saying – this is too hard, why is it taking so long? When it is going to stop? I can't bear this!' I asked her if she would like to invite that part to join the part that is welcoming the baby to be born and see what happens. I watched her as she consciously changed her attention and focus, her demeanour altered and her self talk changed to a heartfelt 'welcome baby'. This is an example of the ego being in the service of the inner self. It did not surprise me when, within twenty minutes, her baby and placenta were born.

EXPANDED ETHICS FOR MIDWIFERY GUARDIANSHIP

When we trained as nurses and midwives (in the 1960s and early 1970s) the institution looked after most ethical issues by defining and enforcing boundaries between nurse and patient; midwife and woman. We were actively discouraged from developing a relationship of any kind, even a professional one. Now, with the new midwifery, all that has changed and we are encouraged to form professional friendships with women and their families that last nearly a year. These relationships involve talking about the most intimate aspects of a woman's life; love, sex, fear, pain, hope, joy and grief. In a midwifery partnership, as described by Karen Guilliland and Sally Pairman (1995), sharing isn't a monologue but a dialogue that involves the midwife sharing something of herself in the process. A midwifery ethics is different from nursing or biomedical ethics (Thompson 2004). The ethical aspects of the relationship between women and midwives come to a crescendo in labour and birth during which many women will experience non-ordinary states of consciousness. During non-ordinary states the woman is extraordinarily vulnerable, sensitive and suggestible requiring a deeper level of self-knowledge and integrity from the midwife.

Inner power and the discernment of good and evil

As Shakespeare famously wrote 'there is nothing either good or bad, but thinking makes it so' (Hamlet, Act 2: Scene 2). When a person accesses the inner self, they find a source of love, wisdom, courage, kindness, strength and power; characteristics we normally label as 'good', they may also encounter fear, anger, hatred and confusion; characteristics we normally label as 'bad'.

The 'inner self' has to rely on wisdom and intuition to discern good from evil, unlike ego which uses rules to justify behaviour. Rules give people direction about what to do in some situations. Rules satisfy the egoic demands for predictability and a false sense of safety; as if learning the rules of behaviour somehow immunizes us from conscious and unconscious unethical behaviour. The problem with following external rules is that one's energy must focus outwards on the rules and in doing that, one loses touch with one's inner self which is the source of 'inner power', wisdom and insight.

Safely accessing the vast reservoir of 'inner power' requires a finely honed ability to discern right from wrong and good from bad. If we are to discern if an attitude, belief or action is in the highest interest of the 'self', there is one question that needs to be answered with the deepest integrity. Is the situation, attitude, belief or action motivated by 'love' or 'fear'? More simply we might ask ourselves; am I moving towards something that I perceive as good (love) or away from something that I perceive as bad (fear)? When we are acting from 'love', our mind–body–spirit is in right relationship.

Love relates to integrative power and serves our highest good. With the exception of life-threatening emergencies, fear is not a reliable motivator for ethically good action. Acting or failing to act based solely on fear, often leads to complications and even chaos. Fear, and its associated stress hormones, causes us to shut down and pull back our energy, which is disintegrative of mind–body–spirit. When we feel fearful, it is time to question what is going on inside ourselves or within a situation. When discerning the answer to these questions, we need to think about whether the attitude, belief or action is in our own highest interests, taking into account the predicted short, medium and long-term consequences for our whole self and all other people in and affected by the situation.

In our view, the professional ethical codes and codes of conduct are not fully adequate for midwifery practice. The codes work well with our egos; they tell us when we have broken a rule. The codes have nothing to offer about how to recognize when we are unconsciously getting into difficult ethical situations. In order to be able to deal with whatever occurs in the woman–midwife partnership the midwife cannot depend upon an external source of knowing what is right and wrong: the midwife needs to be able to discern goodness from within her own 'inner self'. This need, for an inner ethical compass, is even more imperative when the woman and midwife traverse the uncharted territories of non-ordinary consciousness.

Conditions for nurturing ideal midwives

The first step towards ethical relationships is for the midwife, and ideally, the woman, to know and nurture themselves within her own family and community. If the midwife doesn't know or accept herself and/or lacks clear boundaries, then it is likely that her unresolved life issues, her fears and desires will become powerfully entangled with the woman's and/or the woman's partner's fears and desires. Knowing oneself means that the midwife engages in self-exploration and healing by some practice that involves the experience of non-ordinary states of consciousness; e.g. gestalt therapy, bodywork, dreamwork, music therapy, guided hypnosis, breathwork and/or meditation. Accepting yourself means being self-compassionate and self-forgiving. It isn't really possible to authentically offer these gifts to the women in your care unless you begin with yourself (see Box 3.1). A clinical supervisor or professional partner with

whom midwives can discuss their innermost thoughts, fears and desires is also an important safeguard against unethical behaviour.

Ethics for deep and continuing relationships

The deep and continuing woman–midwife relationship calls on us to practise midwifery more consciously. Taking full responsibility for our practice demands a professional framework for understanding the dynamics that occur in professional caring relationships. Some key terms from counselling need to be defined before considering matters of professional ethics in the care of childbearing women. For midwives who want to consistently act from deep personal integrity, Kylea Taylor, a holotrophic breathwork therapist has written on ethics for healers, clergy, therapists and bodyworkers. The ethics that Taylor presents are particularly appropriate for work with women during non-ordinary states of conscious. In the section below we provide a summary and overview of her main ideas as they apply to midwives caring for women in non-ordinary states.

Boundaries: creating a safe container for ethical work

Having clear and unambiguous boundaries creates a safe container for the woman and the midwife to work together. Dealing ethically with boundary issues includes discussing the purpose of the relationship including managing expectations about what the midwife will or will not provide. Reciprocity in the relationship is important so the woman and midwife need to

---

Box 3.1 Midwives need to start with self-nurturing

The most important way a midwife can provide sustainable and ethical professional love is for her to love herself. This means she should look after herself. If you are a midwife, you need to make sure that you are loved and that your needs are met. Consider the following forms of self-love. Read positive self-enhancing books. Nurture your friendships and spend time with positive, life-affirming people. Dedicate time and energy to loving and being loved by your significant others. Make a plan to regularly and frequently enjoy sensuous touch and sex with the one you love or as self-love. Schedule an hour a day for yourself and at least an hour a week in nature. Enjoy the preparation, cooking, presentation and eating of food. Each night, bring to mind three things that you are grateful for from the day; feel the gratitude in your body. Take pleasure in having enough regular sleep. Exercise regularly but make sure it is enjoyable so you will keep it up. Explore yoga, Tai Chi, the martial arts and dancing. Hum and sing often. Play and/or listen to music that reaches your 'inner self'. Learn drumming. Have periodic massages, preferably in silence, where you can let yourself relax completely.

explore and agree what the woman is responsible for and what she will do on her own behalf. Other important matters have to do with negotiating touch, including possible vaginal examinations and touching of breasts. Consent, truth telling and confidentiality need to be discussed. Managing time and money, including issues of professional liability insurance should be openly discussed. The role and scope of the midwife's safe practice should be known to the woman including professional reporting requirements concerning children at risk or in situations of abuse. Midwives are cautioned to avoid providing professional care for a woman with whom you have a close personal relationship. In all the ethical codes, a dual relationship is said to exist between client and professional in which the professional interacts with the client in social, familial, business, political, religious or other contexts which is beyond the professional role (Taylor 1995). Because dual relationships cross boundaries, there is increased potential for ethical violation.

Transference

Transference 'is that set of ways of perceiving and responding to the world which is developed in childhood which is inappropriately transferred into the adult environment' (Peck 1993). As an adult, the woman needs to re-consider her ideas and beliefs from childhood. Becoming an adult means taking responsibility for meeting one's own needs and for making one's own decisions. Transference is the woman's attempt to have the midwife meet the woman's needs directly or take responsibility for the woman's decisions (Taylor 1995). See for example Daphne's story on pg 26.

Transference is a serious matter because, by engaging in this, the woman undermines her own psycho-spiritual process and limits her own potential growth. Transference displaces the woman's self as the site of knowledge and power in her own life. Transference de-rails the woman's potential for spiritual emergence with its accompanying benefits for her transition to motherhood. When transference occurs, or is at risk of occurring, a clear and conscious midwife with good boundaries does not take on the transference no matter how attractive that would be to the midwife's ego. The conscious

midwife reflects the woman's process back to her. For example instead of giving advice when the woman asks you for advice you can help the woman think through what she already knows, what options she has and provide her with non-biased information that she may require in order to make her own decision. Or, if a woman thinks you are an angel because the birth went so well, you can reflect on her strength and inner wisdom in birthing unaided. The best protection when encouraging and supporting the woman engaging in transference is that the midwife abides by the ideal conditions described above.

Counter transference

Counter transference is the inappropriate transference of the midwife's childhood ways of perceiving and responding to the world into the adult world of the woman–midwife relationship. Intense and profound experiences of the woman can trigger unconscious emotions, needs, fears and desires in the midwife which may lead to counter transference. In counter transference the midwife inappropriately, and usually unconsciously, attempts to have his/her unmet needs met by the client (Taylor 1995). Sometimes, because of our own needs to feel powerful, cherished or admired, midwives seek out the role of rescuer, controller or expert in the woman's life.

Example of counter transference in midwifery

Christine

Christine referred to the women she was primary midwife for as 'my girls'. Her 'girls' would only see Christine for antenatal visits. No one else would do. If Christine was up all night with someone having a baby and wasn't there when they came for their scheduled appointment, they wouldn't accept the alternate midwife but would be angry and say they would ring her to make another time. Christine was always being rung by 'her girls' and she even got phone calls late at night about anything from a mother wanting to talk about her baby who hadn't had a bowel action that day to a woman who had a show at 10 am that morning and forgot to tell her. Christine would do all the education for her 'girls' as they didn't want to go to the education sessions run by the midwifery team. Christine always seemed to be on when her 'girls' were in labour and her hours were

Christine   Continued

always far in excess of her allocated hours. Both Christine and her 'girls' were devastated if Christine missed the birth of their babies.

If her partner rang up at work, Christine would be worried that he was angry and that she would be 'in for it' when she got home. Christine never found time to exercise and her eating habits included fast foods and snacks. She began to put on weight and her mood became depressed. Christine seemed to be always complaining about something and her workmates often found it hard to be around her. However, Christine was kindness itself to 'her girls' and never shared with them how she was really feeling.

When the time came for discharge from the midwifery service, both the women and Christine were sad. The women didn't know how they are going to cope without Christine. Christine feels good that the women appreciate her so much and feels it validates her as a midwife and as a good person.

Example of clear and healthy boundaries in midwifery

Joanna

Joanna was passionate about sailing as well as her midwifery work. She and her husband were regular entrants in various sailing races. Joanna loved her time sailing with her husband and organized her workload around spending time with him. When seeing a pregnant woman for her first visit, Joanna spent a lot of time going through the way the midwifery service worked, paying attention to explaining on call rosters, rights and responsibilities of both women and midwives and the guidelines for referral and consultation. Joanna explained that even though she will make every effort to be there for their scheduled antenatal visits, births are unpredictable so it is important for everyone to be flexible and willing to see other midwives if ever she was unavailable. She made sure the women for whom she was primary midwife had at least one visit with the other midwives.

Joanna was very encouraging of the women going to the educational sessions held by all the midwives in the practice (thus reducing the risk of dependency). The women allocated to Joanna readily accept the other midwives as their caregiver at birth if Joanna is off.

Joanna really liked being there when any of the women allocated to her gave birth, but she was just as delighted when the women told her how happy they were with their experience with another member of the team. Joanna gave herself regular massage treats and ensured she did some daily exercise. She was a Pilates and Yoga enthusiast and was good at encouraging women to obtain regular exercise as part of their daily activities. Good nutrition was important for Joanna and she inspired her colleagues and the women to adopt good nutritional habits as well. Joanna never spent more time at work than she needed to, although she could be relied upon to meet her various administrative responsibilities. In the postnatal period, the women often talk and act as if Joanna was at the birth; they forget that she wasn't actually there. Their discharge from the midwifery service is a joyful affair and the women say how happy they are and how much they love their babies and how their relationship with their partner has deepened through this experience. The women don't say that they couldn't have done it without her (Joanna). They feel like they did it themselves.

Carer vulnerabilities to ethical misconduct

Kylea Taylor (Taylor 1995) has developed a model for examining client and caregiver vulnerabilities to ethical misconduct which, for our purposes, is particularly useful for considering issues of counter transference. The reader is strongly encouraged to read Taylor's book as only a sketch of what she wrote can be given here. Taylor's model (Fig. 3.1) is based on the Yogic chakra system and the Buddhist concept of 'right relationship'. There are said to be seven chakras which are subtle energy centres that correspond to the physical nerve plexes of the body. A central energy channel, located 'in the spine threads together these subtle energy centres' (Taylor 1995). At various times in our lives the kundalini energy awakens in the base of the spine and begins its journey upwards towards the crown of the head where pure consciousness is said to await. As the energy becomes active within and between the chakra centres, the person experiences a process of physical and emotional cleansing accompanied by spiritual development or inner transformation and possible external transformation as well. Taylor notes that

Personal fears and spiritual fears		Personal desires and spiritual longings
	7 Oneness	
Fear of losing self-identity Fear of losing God as *Other*		Longing for union Longing for transcendence
	6 Insight	
Fear of seeing things as they are Fear of losing denial Fear of misusing spiritual powers		Longing for mystical understanding Longing for psychic powers Desire to understand the therapeutic process
	5 Truth	
Fear of punishment Fear of criticism Fear of responsibility Fear of being unmasked		Longing to be a conduit for spiritual truth Desire to speak and act with integrity Desire to be free of convention
	4 Love	
Fear of intimacy Fear of separation, abandonment Jealousy		Longing for spiritual connection Longing to be compassionate Desire for openheartedness Desire to be cherished
	3 Power	
Fear of losing control Fear of misusing power Fear of having no effect		Longing to be a healer Desire to control client's process Desire for client's respect Desire for status
	2 Sex	
Fear of transformative energy Fear of touching Fear of sexual contact		Longing for regenerative energy Longing for physical expression, connection Desire for physical touch Desire for sexual contact
	1 Money	
Fear of change Fear of insufficiency		Longing for the unchangeable Longing to embody spirit Need for safety, protection Desire for security Desire for change

Figure 3.1 Caregiver vulnerabilities to ethical misconduct. Adapted with permission from Taylor K 2003 The ethics of caring: Honoring the web of life in our professional healing relationships. Hanford Mead, Santa Cruz.

professional codes of ethics generally focus on ethical misconduct related to the first three chakras: money, sex and power, whereas her model encompasses these but adds love, truth, insight and oneness.

Taylor's concept of 'Right Relationship' is a synthesis of the Buddhist Noble Eightfold Path. The word 'right' connotes appropriateness, love and truthfulness, rather than perfection or the opposite of some arbitrary 'wrong' (Taylor 1995). The Eightfold Path concerns freeing ourselves from fears and desires by attention to in

each of these areas of our life: right understanding, right thought, right speech, right action, right livelihood, right effort, right mindfulness and right concentration.

Essentially the model describes and predicts the form of ethical misconduct that the midwife is vulnerable to because of her unconscious fears, jealousies, desires and longings. Taylor notes that the movement of energy through the chakra centres of the client and the midwife is not always linear. In her model, 'the issues of several centres may be active in any given therapeutic relationship without regard to linearity' (Taylor 1995). Taylor devotes a chapter per chakra which in each case includes a list of questions for self-reflection. These questions are useful when the midwife feels that 'the therapeutic relationship is off-track – somewhere between non-productive and harmful – but is mystified as to where it veered off course' (Taylor 1995). We outline just one chakra and highlight how the vulnerabilities of midwives can create the conditions for unethical conduct.

Ethical vulnerabilities related to love The fourth chakra is where the person moves beyond issues to do with the separate identities. We all long for transcendence beyond the constrictions of money, sex and power issues which are exemplified by the first three chakras. The fourth chakra is about love and the opening of the heart. 'The heart easily enfolds another's joys and sorrows within itself' (Taylor 1995). When a woman is experiencing fourth chakra love there is a sense of sacredness; she just 'being' rather than 'doing' anything. 'She feels a sense of connection to herself, to her caregiver, to nature and to everything she contemplates' (Taylor 1995). In an effective woman–midwife relationship 'the boundaries must be sufficiently well-defined so that both hearts feel enough permission and protection to remain open' (Taylor 1995).

The midwife whose heart is not open, when a women is experiencing an opening of her heart, may long to feel what the woman feels but not be able to. She may feel jealous of the woman's love, ecstasy and serenity. Unconsciously, her jealousy may interfere with the woman's process by; for example, disrupting the loving relationship between the woman and her partner, prematurely cutting the cord during the baby's birth, removing the baby for 'checking' or interfering with breastfeeding. In circumstances like these the midwife's 'own constriction may close in upon the expansive, unfolded and vulnerable heart of the client experiencing love' (Taylor 1995). In writing this we remember times in the past that we have done these things unconsciously. It is important for us and for you to be self-forgiving and self-compassionate about our lack of consciousness at the time and the extent to which we were not living in the ideal conditions (above) to be midwife guardians.

Alternatively the woman's outpouring of love and intimacy, particularly if it occurs when the woman is in a non-ordinary state of consciousness, may fall on the parched earth of the midwife's unfulfilled needs for love. The woman's love is a spiritual form of love (the Greek word agape describes this love) for herself and her baby and possibly her partner. But the midwife 'may feel nurtured by the client's ability to merge, feel and appreciate her unique qualities' (Taylor 1995). The midwife may confuse the woman's spiritual love for her as personal love such as found in ordinary relationships. Indeed, the woman may become confused herself and think that what she experienced in a non-ordinary state was personal love for the midwife. The caregiver can, by sensitively setting appropriate boundaries, help to keep the woman's spiritual love on its correct channel which is within the woman and/or the mother/baby dyad.

When the midwife senses that she is having difficulties with chakra four issues she may consider asking herself some deep questions. Questions such as these are best considered in dialogue with a clinical supervisor or trusted wise colleague. Alternatively you could use journalling as a way of having an honest dialogue with yourself about your relationship to love.

CONCLUSION

This chapter has explored midwifery guardianship as a way of allowing space for the sacred in birthing. Building on the previous chapter where the theory of birth territory was introduced, this chapter continued the theoretical development of the concepts 'integrative' and 'disintegrative power'. Niki's birth story gave an example of how integrative and disintegrative power operates in childbirth.

Within the context of a discussion of spirituality there was a fuller exploration of the notion of 'inner self' and 'inner power' as differentiated from the notion of 'ego' and 'egoic power'. The distinctions between when egoic power is dominating and when egoic power is in the service of the inner self was presented. The healing potential of holotrophic non-ordinary states of consciousness was discussed. The importance of being able to recognize and support women in mild and deep states of non-ordinary consciousness was considered. Finally, the ethics of caring for women during non-ordinary states of consciousness was considered. Particular emphasis was placed on avoiding transference and counter transference because they can derail a woman's spiritual emergence from the childbearing year as a stronger, wiser and more loving person and mother. There is no easy answer to know what the highest good is in many situations because there are so many competing interests. When the midwife feels ethically challenged, if at all possible, she should make decisions after consultation with trusted others who can help her discern the highest good for all concerned based on answering the question 'is this option based on love, including self-love?'

References

Berry Brazelton T 1983 Infants and mothers: differences in development. Dell, New York.

Bourguignon E 1973 Religion, altered states of consciousness and social change. Columbus Ohio State University.

Fahy K, Parratt J 2006 Birth territory: A theory for midwifery practice. Women and Birth 19(2): 45–50.

Goleman D 2003 Destructive emotions and how to overcome them: A dialogue with the Dali Lama. Bloomsbury, London.

Green JV, Coupland et al 1990 Expectations, experiences, and psychological outcomes of childbirth: A prospective study of 825 women. Birth 17(1): 15–24.

Grof S, Grof C 1989 Spiritual Emergency: When personal transformation becomes a crisis. St Martin's Press, New York.

Grof C 1993 The thirst for wholeness: Attachment, addiction and the spiritual path. Harper Collins, San Francisco.

Grof S 1985 Beyond the brain: Birth, death and transcendence in psychotherapy. State University of New York Press, New York.

Guilliland K, Pairman S 1995 The midwifery partnership. Victoria University, Wellington.

Jung CG 1960 On the nature of the psyche. Princeton University Press, Princeton.

Khor G 2004 Reflections on Qi: Tuning your life to the world's hidden energy. New Holland, Sydney.

Kitzinger S 1978 Women as mothers. Martin Robertson, Oxford.

Kornfield J 2002 A path with heart: The classic guide through the perils and promises of spiritual life. Random House, London.

Lahood G 2007 Rumour of angels and heavenly midwives: Anthropology of transpersonal events and childbirth. Women and Birth 20(1).

Lipton B 2005 The biology of belief. Elite Books, Santa Rosa.

Maslow A 1964 Religions, values and peak experiences. Ohio State University Press, Columbus.

Mauger B 1998 Songs from the womb: Healing the wounded mother. Sci Print, Shannon.

Moore B 2004 The Australian Oxford dictionary, 2nd edn. Oxford University Press Online B. Moore. Oxford

University Press, Oxford. http://www.oxfordreference.com.library.newcastle.edu.au:80/views/ENTRY.html?subview=Main&entry=t157.e14252>.

Parratt J 1993 The experience of survivors of incest. Midwifery 10(1): 26–39.

Paul L, Paul B 1975 The Maya midwife as ritual specialist: A Guatemalan case. American Ethnology 2(3): 707–726.

Peck MS 1993 The road less travelled: A new psychology of love, traditional values and spiritual growth. Hutchinson, London.

Schore A 2002 The neurobiology of attachment and early parenting. Republished from Journal of Prenatal and Perinatal Psychology and Health 16(3) B Psychology http://www.birthpsychology.com/birthscene/ppic2.html Accessed 15 December 2006.

Siegal D 1999 The developing mind: How relationships and the brain interact to shape who we are. Guilford Press, New York.

Taylor K 1994 The breathwork experience: Exploration and healing in nonordinary states of consciousness. Hanford Mead, Santa Cruz.

Taylor K 1995 The ethics of caring: Honouring the web of life. Hanford Mead, California.

Thompson F 2004 Mothers and midwives: The ethical journey. Elsevier Science, London.

Walsh D 2006 Subverting the assembly-line: Childbirth in a freestanding birth centre. Social Science and Medicine 62(6): 1330–1336.

Chapter **4**

Territories of the self and spiritual practices during childbirth

Jennifer A. Parratt

'The contraction came and everyone was pushing with me. The baby shot out and into Martin's arms. He scooped her... into my arms and suddenly I was looking at her. We did it... It was a shock to feel something invisible inside and then to be faced with the reality of it...Heidi was really calm. She cried taking her first breath then looked around the room at everyone... Martin was crying and I was crying. It was beautiful... I felt bliss, instantly I forgot all the pain, it was worth it... There was all this cuddling and celebration and absolute happiness. It is difficult to put it into words; there were circles of beautiful energy that connected us all... [Now, nearly 4 months later] I feel like that song "I am woman hear me roar", I feel I can conquer the world! It feels fantastic to have gone through that and to know that I can do it. It's made me see that I can endure a lot more physical pain than I thought I could.' (Jane's story, in Parratt 2005, pp. 11–13)

INTRODUCTION

The focus of this chapter is on the woman within her birth territory. It considers the ordinary changes that women undertake to actualize their potential power to give birth in unique and personally meaningful ways such as that illustrated by Jane, above. Chapter 3 introduced childbirth as having spiritual characteristics that impact on how women experience birth. A specific link was made in that chapter between transcendental peak spiritual experiences and the nonordinary conscious states that women often experience during childbirth. This chapter does not exclude such experiences but also acknowledges that the spiritual ramifications of childbirth extend way beyond the birth room (Gaskin 1990). Based on research exploring the intimate and often ordinary changes that women experience during pregnancy and birth, the chapter considers the ordinary practices of life that encircle childbirth as a peak spiritual experience (Parratt 2008). I call these practices, 'spiritual practices'.

The chapter is in three parts. The first part briefly considers current practices surrounding childbirth change. Part two outlines background concepts to the theory. The final part offers a portion of the theory called 'Territories of the Self' developed from PhD research where 14 women were interviewed in their first pregnancies (Parratt 2008). I re-interviewed the same women twice more in the nine months after the birth. Extracts of the de-identified stories that the women and I jointly constructed are given in this final part of the chapter (Parratt 2005).

'Territories of the Self' embraces the diversity of women as 'embodied selves' (Parratt 2008). 'Embodied self' is a concept that communicates the all-encompassing activity of living undertaken by people; it is indivisible from consideration of our existence as spiritual beings (Irigaray 2001). 'Territories of the Self' uses the word 'territory' in a similar manner to 'Birth Territory' (Fahy and Parratt 2006). Any territory is considered to comprise a physical terrain over which some jurisdiction or power is claimed (Trumble and Stevenson 2002). 'Territories of the Self' refers to the various physical manifestations of the 'embodied self' as well as the inner and outer powers vying for jurisdiction over that self. The contrasting ways that jurisdiction is experienced by an individual 'embodied self' are illustrated in part three with the two concepts, 'spiritual territories' and 'owned territories'.

Although the focus in this chapter is women at birth, it is relevant to us all because we are all 'embodied selves'. An awareness of 'Territories of the Self' highlights the importance of spiritual practices during childbirth by both the woman and the midwife. Spiritual practices teach us to maintain a sense of connectivity and integration despite the disconnections of change. These practices focus on the tiny, apparently insignificant processes of change while also respecting more broadly intended outcomes. When such practices are undertaken,

the woman is most likely to gather her potential, use her power and place herself in the position to experience the best possible, uniquely individual birth appropriate to that particular moment of her life.

CHILDBIRTH CHANGE

This section considers how personal forms of transformation relate to childbirth. It outlines rites of passage theory and contrasts the socially sanctioned rituals with the rituals of familiarity and uniqueness that guide women through the social and personal transformations of childbirth. *Non*rational knowing and power is introduced and the chapter describes how it is misinterpreted and used politically when it is associated with natural birth. The section identifies that being aware of *non*rationality and the on-going intimate changes during childbirth are linked to a sense of integrated wholeness during and after childbirth.

Rites of passage

In general, when considering childbearing, the personal elements of change are bypassed to focus on the overall, more socially evident aspects of the process. The birth process itself is not usually recognized to have transformative qualities although pregnancy and childbirth are recognized as parts of the rites of passage that enable the social transition to motherhood (Davis-Floyd 2003). Rites of passage are the rituals that alter social and self-perceptions in such a way that the person can be perceived to have changed socially (van Gennep 1960; Turner 1972; Davis-Floyd 2003). Rites of passage occur in three broad steps (Davis-Floyd 2003). First is a separation, a disconnection or a sense of not fitting the social norm in some way. Second, this sense of disconnection creates a confusing in-between or 'liminal' state where the person repeatedly becomes aware of not fitting the old or new social positions (Turner 1972). Third, the transformation is completed when the changed self integrates into a new social role.

The liminal phase repeatedly challenges individuals to change. The individual is gradually pressured to release old boundaries of the self which can result in an openness and vulnerability to social suggestions or coercions. Liminality can therefore be perceived as a socially danger-ous state as the individual is open to influences other than those deemed socio-culturally appro-priate (Turner 1972; Davis-Floyd 2003). In addi-tion, the individual can experience liminality as personally dangerous or threatening because it involves the release of socially safe ways of being (Kristeva 1982). A set of rituals that are com-monly known and believed to be necessary can provide a sense of order and predictability for the individual faced with the in-between maze of liminality. A ritual is a 'patterned, repetitive, and symbolic enactment of a cultural belief or value' with the main purpose of transformation (Davis-Floyd 2003, p. 8). By conforming to the socio-cultural values specific to the particular change process the individual's sense of social security is ensured (van Gennep 1960; Davis-Floyd 2003). An example of a socially sanctioned path through liminality is when women enter pregnancy and give birth under the auspice of institutionalized childbirth practices.

Socially sanctioned rituals

Institutionalized childbirth practices form the socially sanctioned rituals that map a linear course from non-pregnant woman, through liminality, to the socially sanctioned role of mother. These insti-tutionalized practices can occur in any setting, not necessarily within the physical walls of an institution. The various predetermined and habit-ually performed practices, whether medical or midwifery, are the socially sanctioned rituals (Davis-Floyd 2003). In this institutionalized birth territory the expert, whether midwife or doctor, is bestowed with a sacred status through specialized knowledge and power (Davis-Floyd 2003 and Chapter 1). The expert applies their knowledge and power from a purely rational perspective whereby the expert considers the woman's knowl-edge and power to be solely sited in her mind (Parratt and Fahy 2008). This is rational dichot-omous thinking, which is biased toward one or other side of a dichotomous pair. Rational thinking also considers the dichotomy absolute and certain, mutually exclusive, and collectively exhaustive (Grosz 1994, 1995). Using rational dichotomous thinking: the woman's knowledge is by definition 'less' than the experts'; expert

knowledge and power is the ultimate resource for all situations; and there is no other rational form of knowledge or power available to the woman.

By using this rational perspective the socially sanctioned childbirth rituals reinforce the order and predictability of science and technology as an essential external reference point for the woman during childbirth change (Davis-Floyd 2003). While women may perceive personal bodily forms of knowledge and power, to the rational thinker these are deemed irrational and a risk to the baby (Parratt and Fahy 2008). Like her caregivers, the woman rationalizes the safety of habitually applied practices over anything that she may personally perceive as more appro-priate. This means her body becomes as much a physiological object to her as it is to the experts.

The overall intention of socially sanctioned rituals is to guide the woman into, through and out of the liminality of childbearing to the socially desired outcome of a physiologically healthy baby with mother as primary caregiver (Davis-Floyd 2003). This socially guided outcome does resonate with women's personal power in the role of mother in the rationalized social world (Davis-Floyd 2003). However, it does so with the rationalized assumption that by guaranteeing this physiological outcome, the overall wellbeing of the woman and baby will be ensured (Parratt and Fahy 2008). Yet, significant numbers of women who conform to the socially sanctioned rituals and give birth using the external power and knowledge of the experts experience dimin-ished wellbeing in the short, medium and long term (Brown and Lumley 1998; Johanson et al 1993; Thompson et al 2002; Borders 2006). This long-term disintegration of women's personal sense of wellbeing impacts on family health and relationships (Boath et al 1998; DeJudicibus and McCabe 2002; Beck and Driscoll 2005). Although the rite of passage to motherhood may be socially fulfilled by the live baby and a nominal woman as mother, the socially sanctioned rituals also serve to disconnect the woman from awareness of an inner sense of her personal change and power.

Rituals of familiarity and uniqueness

In contrast to using socially sanctioned rituals as the guide through liminality, more individually appropriate rituals may be used. These rituals, rather than being focused on order and predictability, focus on familiarity and on individual uniqueness. For example, the familiar sights and sounds of home or the known face of her midwife might be the rituals that create a sense of stability and comfort for the woman. With the sense of security afforded by these familiar rituals the woman can feel free to experience the individual changes of childbirth as special and unique. The woman enacts these rituals in relationship to the contractions of labour which creates a rhythmic oscillating effect: as the woman releases bodily control, she relinquishes mental focus; then further releases bodily control and so on (Parratt and Fahy 2003). She can gain a sense of the familiar through this rhythmic repetition yet the positions, movements and timing of these practices are uniquely hers.

Birth territories that enable these individually appropriate rituals are experienced as perceptibly safe to the woman, rather than merely rationalized as safe regardless of how the woman feels (Parratt and Fahy 2004, 2008). In perceptibly safe birth territories midwives responses are open and fluid so as to allow for the individual diversity of each woman and each situation (Klassen 2001). The fluidity of midwifery responses to each labouring women is, in part, why such an incredible diversity of spiritual experiences have been identified during childbirth (Klassen 2001). Responsivity to women as unique individuals enables midwives to honour both women's capability of giving birth naturally and at the same time apply individually appropriate, holistic intervention when required (Downe and McCourt 2004). It is this focus on the particularities of the individual woman that can enable each woman to undertake her own ordinary practices that lead her to find the power within herself to give birth.

These perceptibly safe birth territories move beyond the linear overall change of socially sanctioned rituals; they embrace a second more cyclical form of inner change which can be symbolized by the rhythmic oscillations of labour. In perceptibly safe birth territories the oscillating relationship between rituals of familiarity and uniqueness continually assist the woman to create and recreate her own particular sanctum in which to give birth. Through her overall

linear progress toward the birth but also in the cyclical intimacy of moment to moment change, the rituals of familiarity and uniqueness push the woman to find a sense of knowledge and power within herself. Then, via this free flow of inner power, the aim of labour is transformed into the actuality of birth. This inner power intimately transforms the woman as the birth is occurring. The power also works to transform her identity after the birth in the daily activity of living.

Nonrational power and knowing

*Non*rationality is all the embodied ways of knowing and experiencing that are beyond rational, dichotomous thought and language. Women may experience inner power as a connecting force to their baby, their body or their god (Klassen 2001). The extract from Jane's story at the beginning of this chapter illustrates her experience of inner power and knowledge. She feels herself as an integrated whole who is also part of the larger whole that is her world, yet the birth is an experience of separation too. She releases her baby from her body to socially transform to mother, and she disconnects from pain and worry to experience a self-transformation. It is an enormous release for her that changes her perception as it connects and energizes her with regard to herself, her baby and those around her.

Jane's birth experience is intimately and inexpressibly meaningful to her. Even four months after the birth, Jane still experiences a related sense of power and knowing. When using rational dichotomous thinking, these experiences are labelled 'irrational' and ignored as irrelevant or linked to a sense of madness or badness (Parratt and Fahy 2008). However, rather than being irrational, inner power and knowing is *non*rational, because it is a very real experience, yet is difficult to explain using rational language (Kovel 1991). The *non*rational aspects of life can be described as mysterious, sacred, spiritual, intuitive and experientially grounded. Such experiences are part of the fullness of our lives as integrated whole 'embodied selves' diversely interacting in the world.

During women's experience of childbirth, midwives also have the capacity to change and become aware of *non*rational power and knowing. The midwife may be particularly aware of this when intuitive powers are drawn on in addition to more rational forms of practice (Davis-Floyd and Davis 1997). Being open to the *non*rational at birth can teach midwives about trust, courage and their own intuitive abilities (Roncalli 1997). When the *non*rational at each birth is honoured, midwives have the opportunity to be reminded of the inherent ability of women to undertake the functions of life, healing and birth without standard technological manipulations (Roncalli 1997). No matter what level of past experience the midwife has had, each birth can prompt a degree of transformation for the midwife as well as for the woman.

Empowerment and natural birth

Although a sense of the *non*rational tends to be difficult to relay in words, the feelings of integrated wholeness that result from such experiences can promote a desire to share them through language. Stories of *non*rational power are therefore often used to give voice to birth experiences in the public domain and to teach midwives (Pairman et al 2006; Vernon 2006). However, these words often do more than share a personal experience of empowerment; they have an underlying intention to empower others. In the context of childbirth, the intention to empower others has been called the 'spiritualizing of homebirth'; it powers much of the natural birth movement (Klassen 2001, p.73).

Having arisen from the 1970s feminist movement where women wished to be freed from the regimes of institutionalized birth, the natural birth movement is not only espoused by women who actually experience natural birth. Midwives have also desired freedom from medically directed birth, so they have taken on a role of empowering women toward natural birth (Brown 2003). As a result, the ideology of empowerment has become identified as an acceptable and valuable measure of satisfactory childbirth (Harcombe 1999). Entangled in the rhetoric of empowerment is the push for informed choice and control over decision-making. However, empowerment through informed choice is not necessarily a successful strategy, as the provision of information

for decision-making is determined by the power of the person providing that information (Levy 1999). Additionally, the more unilaterally caregivers make decisions, the less empowered women actually feel (Vande Vusse 1999). What is more, empowerment has been used to promote both natural and medical birth (Beckett 2005).

For many people, the concept of natural childbirth provides an immediate symbolic link between birth and the universal capabilities of the female body. However, because of this link to the universal, the concept actually says far more (Beckett 2005). For example, it can be taken to mean that all women want or should want natural birth. Indeed, it can also be taken to mean that all women should want babies so they can experience the power of natural birth. But the most damaging message that the concept of natural birth relays is that at some essential level, all women are the same and therefore, all women can experience childbirth in essentially the same way. Ironically, the message that all women can experience childbirth in the same way also underlies how medicine conceptualizes childbirth (Chapter 1).

Misinterpreting the *non*rational

Positioning the personal experience of *non*rational power in the socio-political arena of natural birth creates the same assumptions and generalizations as used in medicalized birth. This occurs because both natural and medical birth discourses are rational conceptualizations of childbirth. Both discourses conceptualize childbirth in terms of absolutes and certainty. Both claim priority over the other and consider no other options to be equally valid. And both perceive the changes of childbirth in purely linear terms. With these rationalized concepts, the woman's potential during childbirth becomes institutionalized according to the natural or medical boundaries placed around the experience. Arguments about dichotomies such as natural/medical, home/hospital, midwife/doctor, female/male, body/mind, or intuition/reason merely serve as distractions from the experiential reality of childbirth change. The profound nature of experiential reality is lost when personal transformation is translated into social rhetoric via rational means.

Even with the best laid intentions for childbirth, the disconnective changes of liminality can be challenging. When women and caregivers have little experiential grounding in the *non*rational aspects of childbirth change, childbirth change becomes interpreted in a rational, dichotomous manner. Whether the intention is toward natural birth or not, during the actual process of childbirth, an assumption is taken that transformation refers to a single instance of linear change. By seeing only this big picture overview, the focus of the change process is on the end result alone. In ignoring the individual nuances of cyclical change, the labouring woman's opportunities for finding uniquely suited rituals is limited, which then limits her openness to further change. The transforming potential of each one of those cycles of change is therefore missed or subverted by the focus on a desired (or undesired) outcome. The woman and/or midwife is more likely to turn to the habitually chosen practices of socially sanctioned rituals and standard techno-medical means to accomplish the birth.

*Non*rational power is inexpressibly unique, diverse and whole at the experiential level. Conceptualization of the sense of integration that accompanies *non*rational experiences is like a foreign language to a person who has had little experiential awareness of *non*rationality. Retaining a sense of wellbeing during and after childbirth is linked to the embodied sense of integrated wholeness that *non*rational awareness of change can provide. These understandings embrace the individual and unique potential of each individual 'embodied self' experiencing the intimacy of moment to moment cycles of change as they relate inwardly toward the self and outwardly to the world. The next section introduces the spiritual practices and considers the *way* 'embodied self' undertakes ordinary, intimate change as it impacts on whether potential is actualized.

EMBODIED SELF AND THE BOUNDARIES OF POTENTIAL

This section aims to give definition to terms such as 'embodied self', spirit and soul while outlining the boundaries of potential. The paradox of being an integrated whole 'embodied self' while also changing is considered. The section outlines what it means to *be* an 'embodied self' and how rational egoic reflections shape views of *non*rationality. It highlights how a disjunction between intent and action can occur and suggests that choosing spiritual practices can enhance the potential to actualize intention.

Spirit: idiosyncratic and unbounded

'Embodied selves' shape their understanding of spirituality according to the contexts in which they live (Klassen 2001). Religions and spiritual texts offer some structure to what spirituality may be, but personal understandings of spirituality are as diverse as people are diverse. In this chapter I make the assumption that spirituality is inherent in all human existence and I define spirituality as the ways that people become aware of spirit and soul in their lives (Kovel 1991). The experience of spirituality is thus the practices, production and responses to spirit (Kovel 1991).

Spirit is power (Kovel 1991). It animates, inspires and gives vitality. As a power it is ethically neutral (Chapter 1). It acts to create and sustain connections but also to break them. Spirit is *non*rational, ever moving and acts in sometimes idiosyncratic ways as it is free of what we rationalize as possible and impossible. The direction, force and flow of spirit extend beyond rational boundaries of time, space and matter. Without the boundaries that give us a sense of the absolute and certainty, spirit has the potential to change and liberate phenomenon (Kovel 1991). Spirit can be experienced as sacred, mysterious or wondrous; as a passive yielding or surrender; as energy or enthusiasm; as an intuitive gift; or simply as the breath (Kovel 1991).

The power of spirit is the energy underlying all that is in the world and the cosmos; it has been given other names, for example Universal Energy (Chapter 3) and the subtle yet vital energy called *qi* (said 'chee') (Chen 2004). *Qi* is an expression of the absolute and beyond; it is all that can be thought of as well as all that cannot even be imagined. Spirit (*qi*) is symbolized by the Yin Yang pictogram (☯) as the universal law of tao (or dao) which refers to the *way* 'embodied self' exists with planned change as well as unintended change (Tzu 1963; Wilhelm and Baynes 1967).

The pictogram symbolizes spirit's *non*rational wholeness which paradoxically also incorporates dichotomies symbolized as dark and light sides that include part of the light in the dark and part of the dark in the light. It illustrates that everything may be dichotomously paired yet nothing is permanently one or the other as each are relative to the other. The *way* of existence is a reference to the moment to moment choices that 'embodied self' may make to honour (through spiritual practices) or ignore (through habitual practices) these paradoxes.

Spiritual practices

Eastern spiritual practices revolve around the cultivation of spirit (as *qi*) in combination with intention (called *yi*) in the self-practice of 'Qigong' (Chen 2004). In 'Qigong' the meditative practice of intention acts to position mind and body as well as cultivate the spirit through the breath. Yoga is a similar practice of energy management. Intention refers not only to the overall aim that a person may have but also the manner or *way* in which it is enacted (Kovel 1991; Hanh 1995; Lacan 2004). The spiritual practice of intention involves an increase in a person's awareness of even the smallest, most intimately ordinary degrees of change and then acting on it mindfully (Hanh 1995). Mindfulness is a spiritual practice that promotes: a sense of whether or not one's choices and aims are free of manipulation by the self or others; a decrease in materialist desires; and the implementation of unconditional love through forgiveness, trust and acceptance of the self and the world (Hanh 1995). It teaches that any one perception of truth is not the only truth and that intention which is solely based on self-serving goals is not always the best for a person's overall wellbeing (Hanh 1995).

As spirit exists inside and outside our bodies even the spatial arrangement of physical objects, called 'feng shui', can influence its flow and is part of spiritual practice (Curl 2006). Skilled practitioners can even direct their spirit externally to assist the healing of others (Chen 2004). Modern science and medicine have undertaken considerable research in the effects of spirit (as *qi*) on health and healing (Chen 2004). For example there is evidence that the practice of Qigong can positively affect hypertension, asthma, blood viscosity, immunity, serum lipid levels, longevity and the rates of stroke (Sancier and Holman 2004). Although these effects have been demonstrated, it is unclear how the healing occurs. Nonetheless the effects of Qigong do illustrate that spiritual practices can enhance our energy for ordinary existence as 'embodied selves'.

Soul: the ongoing embodiment of spirit

The embodied expression of spirit is the soul (Trumble and Stevenson 2002). Soul is the intimate, candid, all-inclusive breadth and depth of who we are and what we make of ourselves. Soul creates our experiential reality in any particular context and enables a sense of integration within the self as well as between the self and the world (Kovel 1991). The living, breathing entirety of 'embodied self' is the interconnected unity of body, soul and mind within the particular context of life experience.

Soul is indivisible from 'embodied self's' existence but this can lead to a misapprehension of soul as limited by organic existence, perhaps to a particular site in the body such as the heart or the mind. Furthermore, 'embodied self' can interpret experience of the soul in diverse and contrasting ways, for example as good, evil, joyous or sad. However, soul is the organic expression of the *idiosyncratic* connections of spirit. This means that soul moves in parallel with spirit, is ethically neutral, and can cross rational boundaries of time, space and matter (Kovel 1991). Like spirit, the eccentricities of soul can act to integrate and connect as well as to disconnect, divide, change and liberate (Kovel 1991). It is because of this ongoing embodying process of connection and disconnection that we can each be aware of differences within ourself, between ourselves, and over time. The oscillating movement between connection and disconnection means that the 'embodied self' is in a continual state of change relating inwardly and outwardly according to its own particular context at any point of time (Irigaray 1993, 2001; Lacan 2004).

Oscillating relationships: disconnecting and connecting

The circumstances and settings of 'embodied self's' current existence make up its context. Contexts incorporate inwardly sensed feelings, thoughts, desires or memories; they may be outwardly focused to include people and their actions, statements or ideas; they may also encompass the physicality of the body, the bodies of others or other parts of the physical environment. Contexts are ever changing in an oscillating interaction with 'embodied self' and whatever else is in that context. The oscillatory process occurs not only with regard to the animate parts of our environment but to the inanimate aspects as well. Consider how the air we breathe changes between inspiration and expiration. Depending on the context we can seemingly merge, connect, or integrate for a time with parts of our environment in various ways. This integration may be with other people, their ideas, or the tools and technologies of our environment (Haraway 2000; Irigaray 2001; Lacan 2004).

The Yin Yang pictogram (☯) symbolizes the continual movement of an integrated whole 'embodied self' who is also interacting via connections and disconnections with contexts that are themselves ever changing. More broadly, the pictogram illustrates how dichotomies are never totally disconnected but act in a changing relationship with each other. This paradoxical duality is evident in the extract of Jane's story. Jane had physically disconnected from her baby by giving birth yet she also felt a great sense of connection to her babe. These oscillating changes occurring within and without 'embodied self' mean that the 'embodied self' is created and recreated within the contexts of relationships (Robb 2006). Yet despite this continual change 'embodied self' also retains an ongoing potential to sense itself as integrated and whole.

Being and potential

Actual existence as an integrated whole 'embodied self' in the here and now is 'being' (Kovel 1991; Hanh 1995). 'Being' encompasses the wholeness of our experiences: of sexuality; of movement in space and time; of perception and emotion; and even of our *experience* of thought and language (Merleau-Ponty 2002). An instance of 'being' is an in the moment experience that is pre-reflective: it occurs 'prior' to thoughts or responses to it. 'Being' is *non*rational as its sense of integrated wholeness cannot be fully relayed conceptually. An instance of 'being' holds *non*rational knowing and power which differs from any knowing or power derived from the action of reflection that follows. It is the experiential prior knowing of instances of 'being' yet to be (Merleau-Ponty 2002; Wynn 2002). Although it is *non*rational, contemporary physiological research also recognizes the existence of prior knowledge as the information that allows bodies to predict demand and adjust parameters to meet potential needs (Sterling 2004). Each instance of 'being' therefore holds this *non*rational prior knowing which is the potential of other instances of 'being' (Hanh 1995; Kovel 1991).

Potential is a latent form of power that over time will or will not be actualized (Trumble and Stevenson 2002). Potential cannot be held or touched or seen, yet it is always present, even in inanimate objects. In the 'embodied self' the power of potential is *non*rational and indivisible from the soul; it cannot be predicted in rational, linear, cause and effect ways (Wynn 2002). Our souls know the experiential truth of our potential and an experiential awareness of it is expressed as the inner self, inner knowing, inner strength or inner power. Awareness of this experiential knowing can provide courage and security through the changes experienced in ordinary life. Furthermore, the *non*rational power and knowing contained in each instance of 'being' is also a resource to draw on when faced with changes that are beyond the ordinary, such as during childbirth.

Ego and ways of 'being'

The *way* in which 'embodied selves' exist with change is also influenced by the rational, reflective power of the ego. The ego is an entirely embodied power that allows us to reflect on any particular moment of 'being' and make choices about the next way of 'being' (Lacan 1977, 2004; Grosz 1994, 1995). Ego continually makes these choices, most often below the level of awareness. It does this by contrasting, comparing and prioritizing all that our senses, including our mind, tell us about our 'embodied self' and our context. These actions are disconnective and biased towards what ego thinks will keep the self safest. Yet it is through this process we gain perspective on our existence across time (e.g. past and future) and across space (e.g. relating to other people) thereby giving us the capacity to choose particular ways of 'being' and influence the *way* we exist with change.

By using this process the ego creates stable, certain boundaries around the self and the world which often exclude any perspective of the 'embodied self' as changing (Lacan 2004). The texture of 'embodied self's' contexts are continually influenced by these boundaries. While these boundaries may seem very real they are merely reflections derived from ego's biased assessment of experiential reality, they are not experiential reality itself (Lacan 2004). Nonetheless, the experiential reality of 'being' sometimes challenges ego boundaries and creates a disconnective sense of unease or even fear (Lacan 1977, 2004; Kristeva 1982). Sometimes our awareness of this disconnection can dominate to such a degree that a sense of connection (inner or outer) can seem impossible. We can feel ourselves to be alienated, 'split', confused, and divided; by no means an integrated 'embodied self'. Such reminders of the changeability of 'embodied self' threaten ego boundaries so ego works hard to protect against uncertainty, unpleasantness or pain by the embodied storage of ways of 'being' (Lacan 1977, 2004).

A sense of security can arise from these egoic ways of 'being' as they provide boundaries of how to behave in new situations. We can even gain the sense that we own these ways of 'being' because they become the definitional boundaries used to define who we are and who we are not in particular situations; thus, these ways of being are termed the 'owned territories'. However, depending on the *way* in which 'embodied self' chooses to exist, our owned ways of 'being' can also create boundaries around our potential to find new ways of 'being' when parts of our contexts are changing. For this reason, ego's underlying self-protective stance does not necessarily sustain the integrated wholeness of 'embodied self'. Indeed sometimes ego's insistent maintenance of habitual practices can literally be disintegrative to 'embodied self'.

Intention, action and choice

With potential ways of 'being' limited to those that the ego considers rationally possible and

least challenging to its boundaries, we may find ourselves consciously intending one thing while our owned ways of 'being' actually lead us in another direction (Lacan 1977, 2004). This disjunction between intent and action occurs because whether we are aware of it or not, our ego is continually influenced by the *non*rational power of potential. Our *way* of existence is therefore constantly shaped by the ongoing oscillating interaction between ego and potential as symbolized by the alternating sides of the Yin Yang pictogram (☯).

Each time we become aware of experiential change and disconnection we are faced with choice. Do we maintain our habitual practices and allow ego's rationalizations to dominate? Do we disconnect from *non*rational power and undertake ways of being that are disintegrative, making the actualization of potential and the achievement of intention unlikely? Or do we forgive the disconnections that necessarily occur with change? Do we undertake spiritual practices and focus on the connections that continue within our 'embodied self' and/or our context? Do we utilize our ego with humility and recognize its boundaries might be clouding experiential reality? Do we open the definitional boundaries of our ego to the wiles of *non*rational power and act in integration toward a common purpose that actualizes potential and achieves our intention? The next section introduces the spiritual practices of integrative ways of 'being'. These practices can collectively enhance the potential for the actualization of uniquely experienced, personally transforming birth.

PATHWAYS OF POTENTIAL

This section outlines the spiritual practices with regard to disintegrative and integrative ways of 'being'. Table 4.1 presents some of the processes contained within ways of 'being' and the theoretical concepts linked to disintegrative and integrative ways of 'being'. The two ways of 'being' shown in Table 4.1 and illustrated in this section compose only one of the three pathways through change that are encompassed in the whole of 'Territories of the Self' (Parratt 2008). The theory is based on the understanding that the 'embodied self' is ever changing, as is its context and therefore,

Table 4.1   Disintegrative and integrative ways of 'being'

Ways of 'being' – relevant elements (may occur simultaneously)	Potential: Disintegration-concepts	Potential: Integration-concepts
Utilizing power	*Disintegrative power*	*Integrative power*
Power use by self toward self and toward environment. Impact on self of how power is used in environment (also Ch. 3). Influenced by ego boundaries brought into current context.	Action taken to maintain dominance of ego's self protective intention. Ego contrasts, compares and judges potential ways of 'being' using linear, rational dichotomous thinking. Use of other processes to assess ways of 'being' are considered irrational. Promotes conformity to and reliance on prioritized ways of 'being'.	Action taken to adjust ego boundaries so self-protective intentions do not dominate. Prioritized ways of 'being' are released. Ego boundaries soften and open to the potential of *nonrational* ways of 'being' synchronous to specific context. Promotes clarity of overall intention so power is directed to well-being of whole 'embodied self' in current context rather than to ego boundaries.
Responding to change	*Qualified strength*	*Integrated strength*
Ego response to changing 'embodied self' and/or contextual change. Influenced by degree of self-awareness and personal choices (mindfulness).	Ego's rationalized, qualified judgments limit and dominate. Conditional strength accessed by maintaining definition and certainty of ego boundaries.	Ego's inward and outward judgements are open to and integrate with *nonrational* forms of knowing. Unconditional strength accessed by increasing awareness of *non-rational* potential.
Existing experientially	*Owned territories*	*Spiritual territories*
Actual experiential existence in current context. Influenced by degree of mindfulness currently experienced.	Existence experienced according to qualified strength. Encompasses a disconnection from and/or active exclusion of other ways of 'being' according to ego's perception of context.	Existence experienced as irreducible wholeness through inward and outward integration. Encompasses *experiential* awareness of potential. Inclusive of disconnection from and connection to other ways of 'being' according to context currently experienced.
Contributing to outcome	*Forced birth**	*Genius birth**
How ego's input into change creates new ways of 'being'. Influenced by degree of self-awareness and personal choices (mindfulness).	Old ways of 'being' are relatively released. New ways of 'being' arise by being forced into existing ego boundaries resulting in some disintegration of 'embodied self'. Ego boundaries are preserved and perceived impossibilities are confirmed.	Old ways of 'being' are absolutely released making room for new ways of 'being' that are most appropriate to context. Sense of integrated 'embodied self' is preserved. Ego boundaries soften and open enabling what was previously perceived as impossible to become experiential reality.

*With regard to the actual birth experience **genius birth** and **forced birth** may or may not include the use of medico-technology. **Genius birth** represents the activity of an integrated 'embodied self' using her own power to give birth in the best possible, uniquely individual way for that particular woman at that particular moment of her life. **Forced birth** refers to birth that is primarily devoid of spontaneity and contrived to fit the pre-determined boundaries of the woman and/or her attendants.

it is the *way* in which the self changes that impacts on our ability to actualize our potential.

Five extracts from women's stories are used to illustrate these ways of 'being' (Parratt, 2005). These extracts are taken from far longer stories. For clarity I have rearranged some paragraphs more chronologically. I have deleted words which I signify with '...' and where I have added words I place them in square brackets [ ]. I also include interpretive comments that relate each extract to the concepts of 'Territories of the Self'.

Each woman is having her first baby. Jasmin (Parratt 2005, pp. 81–98) and Maree (pp. 119–138) plan for home birth and are transferred to hospital, Emily (pp. 167–188) plans to use a birth centre and is transferred to a standard labour ward, while both Jane (pp. 1–16) and Gina (pp. 99–118) have their babies at home. In these extracts Jasmin tells of how she planned for her birth to go a certain way, Emily worries about whether labour will start, Maree loses the rhythm she finds through labour, Jane needs to share responsibility in order to let go and push, while Gina achieves what seemed impossible and actually does 'it'. Disintegrative ways of 'being' dominate Jasmin's plans, but for each of the other women a change to integrative ways of 'being' makes an impact on their ability to actualize their potential. In the stories below new theoretical concepts are **emboldened**; their definitions can be found in Table 4.1.

Planning a certain way

Jasmin's story

'If I've got a place to go and everything around me that I need, [labour] will be a really positive experience. The only thing I can do is control the environment... I've set myself up really well with support people and two midwives... I've prepared a room specifically... She is being born in her own room in water... My friend Hannah... did a lot of preparation for a natural birth but had a Caesar... she didn't have access to the same level of information about birth as I have.'

Jasmin accesses **qualified strength** to gain security about the birth. She experiences this security as the **owned territories** of being certain about where her baby is to be born. She is so sure of this she uses **disintegrative power** to explain why her friend didn't do what Jasmin is certain she will do. Then in labour:

'I was prepared for letting go...I trusted that the people I needed were in the room and because those supports were around me I was able to give up... control. But Mae [my midwife] became quite ill... and was often out of the room. I couldn't focus during contractions without her. I became scared when I knew a contraction was coming; then the fear developed into... panic... In between contractions I'd have my eyes on Mae whenever she moved... Leanne [my second midwife] was trying to help but... she just

wasn't Mae. My husband tried holding me but I didn't want a bar of that... The minute Mae put her hand on my forehead it was all right, I could do it. I just needed that soothing voice, I was really clinging and in between I was apologizing... [After Mae left and I knew labour was not going to plan] I was panicking, screaming and completely out of control. I didn't have Mae holding my hand, the pool, or that peaceful, everything's going to be all right feeling. I was in free fall; I had no surety [my baby] was going to be born at home, I didn't know what was going to happen...'

Jasmin again accesses **qualified strength** to enable her to let go. But when those strengths are removed she is left to experience the fearful reality of her **owned territories**. In her **owned territories** no one and nothing else will do, she must have her midwife and the birth must go according to her plan.

'Hospital wasn't the big demon that I thought it was going to be... Leanne was with me and I felt quite safe... [but] I still believed I was going to have... a natural birth although I wasn't quite sure how... It was all so hard and out of control... A doctor pressured me saying, "has anyone talked about caesarean"... I was buying time for Mae to tell me I wouldn't need to talk about it; I thought there would be another card in the bag... I had felt completely in control beforehand, it was terrible to have it go so far from the plan I thought I could guarantee myself the best outcome by surrounding myself with the right tools: I studied, did all the possible preparation, and employed my own midwives. I put so much effort into having it go a certain way.'

Jasmin makes little adjustment to her ego boundaries when she takes on new ways of 'being' by accepting the other midwife and going to hospital (**forced birth**). She keeps the experiential security of her owned **territories**, she still accesses **qualified strength** from her midwife and uses **disintegrative power** to maintain the illusions of her ego. Try as she might, she cannot force her birth to go the certain way she planned.

Worrying about whether labour will start

Emily's story

'I really believed that I would go into labour... the whole team of hospital midwives had real faith in me. They suggested things to help me get into labour and said I could ring any time. Even though I had plenty of

Emily's story   Continued

knowledge just knowing they were there was reassuring... [but] as I got more overdue I worried that maybe I was being crazy waiting... I found it very easy to default to that rational part of me... I [even] initiated a conversation about Caesars... but I was... encouraged to be patient...'

Emily initially accesses **integrated strength** from her own belief and from her midwives. But as she is further challenged she reverts to using her rationalized **disintegrative power** and accesses **qualified strength**. Nonetheless her environment (midwives and obstetrician) uses **integrative power** and she is encouraged to be patient.

'I'd been through conversations with myself about why my baby's head was still high... I worried I had talked my body into being overdue because I'd worked until late in pregnancy and nothing was ready... By this point my doubts and fears were so real ... I began to question why I was waiting... I had to stand back and ask myself who I was in the experience and I tried to let my body be.'

Emily continued using **disintegrative** power on herself by worrying over causation and experiencing her **owned territories**. But rather than persisting on this path she begins to use **integrative power** and accesses **integrated strength**. By looking inside herself she increases her awareness of bodily experience in the **spiritual territories**.

'When I was 11 days over I felt petrified because I hadn't had any foetal movements for 3 hours, I thought maybe I'd gone too far and should get induced. I knew if I had been going to a different hospital I'd have been induced that day. I contemplated going to have the heart beat done, but part of me asked what running to someone else was going to achieve. I realized I had to accept whatever was going to come from this, that my body would tell me what was coming. I'd either have more movements or I wouldn't...I didn't leave home; I just squatted outside in the garden, calming my mind and feeling acceptance of my body. The midwives and doctor's faith in me got me up to that point and then faith in myself got me the next three days ...the day before I was due to start Prostin, my membranes ruptured.'

Again Emily is challenged and experiences the fears of her **owned territories**. She contemplates accessing **qualified strength** but instead uses **integrative power** and accesses **integrated strength**

by listening to questions that arise and to her body. She takes courage in the experience of **spiritual territories** and actively uses **integrative power** to allow a new way of 'being' to begin with the **genius birth** of her labour.

Losing the rhythm: starting to push

Maree's story

'Often I almost forgot the image of hospital while I focused on my husband at home feeling pleased and cheering me on... Contractions were fairly full on but didn't take over my body; I felt quite controlled and got into a rhythm of focused letting go... I never really went off into another space although as the contractions increased and got more difficult I needed to put more energy into being centred and focused so I would talk less...Every time a contraction started I would take a big breath in and focus really deeply. All the way through I would sing a low note and visualize a downward movement of him and an outward sound for me. I felt the vibration from the noise I made down the centre of my body giving me the sensation of actually centring internally... The repetitive stuff and familiar things strengthened my centeredness. It was the type of centring where the vibration of the note is far more powerful than all of that chaos going on around me like the pain and my friends talking me through the contractions.'

Maree continually accesses **integrated strength** partially from the positive image of her husband but primarily from within herself. In doing so she experiences the **spiritual territories**. Her use of **integrative power** is an activity focused on the breath, sound vibration and bodily focus that helps her maintain the **spiritual territories** despite distractions.

'[But]...I seemed to lose the rhythm and couldn't get centred any more... my body was pushing... I still had a long way to go so I felt I must need to do a poo and sat on the toilet for 3 or 4 contractions. That's when I lost control. The contractions were coming too quickly to be able to think... [My midwife] was giving me all the advice about interventions I could end up with but I wasn't really being given the option to not take them... Hearing what she said made me doubt whether I could

Maree's story   Continued

physically go on without intervention. . . I was getting quite upset because I couldn't get back to that centred feeling and it was even more painful.'

Maree is secure with the rhythm and centred feeling she has experienced so losing those sensations becomes an experience of the **owned territories**. Her midwife is using **disintegrative power** and they both access **qualified strength** with the assumption that Maree still has a long way to go. Doubt creeps in to her experience of **owned territories** as she continues to miss the sense of being centred.

'It really felt like something needed to come out. . . I was standing up and as the pain came I'd bend over and lift a leg up to try to cope with it. . .I was fully dilated. . . [I sat on] a birth stool. . . and suddenly. . . I didn't feel another contraction. . . [just] that pushing feeling.'

Nonetheless Maree still listens to her body. She returns to using **integrative power** and begins a different experience of **spiritual territories**. She accesses **integrated strength** and creates new ways of 'being'. The **genius birth** of the pushing phase of her labour begins and in due course leads to her baby's birth.

Sharing responsibility and letting go

Jane's story

'Then the urge to push started. . . In first stage I wasn't thinking about what I was doing but now I was conscious of what was happening. . . [it was] a very different feeling. . . I [had] thought. . . the baby would just slip out on its own. When I realized that it wasn't going to I felt really scared. In my mind this baby was huge and it was just bizarre to think it was going to get down this canal. I thought "nothing I'm doing is going to get this baby out". I was shocked by what was expected of me compared to what I'd just gone through.'

Jane accesses **qualified strength**, uses **disintegrative power** and experiences the **owned territories** as she finds herself thinking about what is required to push.

'It was in my control to push but I was scared to do it. . . I didn't have the. . . confidence, the belief and even the desire to do it. It was the lowest point for me; if I had been in the situation where a caesarean

was offered that was the point where I would have said "yes". . . I couldn't see how it was possible for me to push her out. I was focusing on those really negative outcomes, and that wasn't allowing any positive thought. . .I used what little will I did have to slow down that natural urge to push. . .I was fighting against it, tensing up and resisting the push. . .'

Jane's use of **disintegrative power** compromises her power so she has no confidence or desire to push. She keeps her **owned territories** and accesses **qualified strength** with her negative focus and uses **disintegrative power** to resist pushing.

'. . .I was too caught up to ask for help. . . the fear, the lack of confidence, the negative focus and all that impossibility in my head was getting in the way. . .I confessed to [my partner] that I was really scared. I could see he was really anxious; he tried to be supportive but with every contraction I was saying "I can't do it". I chose him because, rather than make me face the fear; I knew he would agree with my beliefs that I couldn't do it. . .I was hiding my fear because telling the midwives would have meant doing what I thought was impossible. . .'

Jane is so determined in her use of **disintegrative power** she avoids the midwives and accesses **qualified strength** from her partner who strengthens the disintegrative ways of 'being' with his own fear thereby maintaining Jane's experience of the **owned territories**.

'But [my midwife]. . .figured out what was going on eventually. . . [she] said "why are you resisting each contraction" and that's when I said I was scared. I felt an enormous responsibility to get the baby out. By guiding me through it [she] took a bit of that responsibility away. . . even though it was still up to me, [my midwife] was ultimately responsible for getting me through it by talking to me. . . Their belief that I could do it made me do it, it brought me into the present, stopped me from being all flighty and worried. It took me out of my head and into my body to what I had to do. . .It was a big relief to stop resisting and finally begin to let go.'

Jane's **owned territories** are based on her fear of responsibility. Once she allows herself to work with the **integrative power** from her midwives and begins to access **integrated strength** her experience moves into the **spiritual territories**. She uses integrative power along with the midwives so that all share responsibility. This integrative approached thus enables Jane to give **genius birth** to new ways of 'being' by letting go.

Actually doing it

> ### Gina's story
>
> *'The whole labour felt like a letting go, but pushing didn't. I was consciously aware of it as a physical activity, something that I had to get in there and do, so to some degree I had to come out of that animalistic letting go phase. I felt that I needed to take control of it but at the same time I knew I had no control either way. Pushing was mostly involuntary but I needed that voluntary mind set...'*
>
> Gina is in the **spiritual territories** during labour and as she becomes aware of the differences required for pushing she maintains the **spiritual territories** by using **integrative power** and accessing **integrated strength**.
>
> *'I was thinking, "you're the only one who can do this", but I said, "I can't do this", and my support people would answer "yes you can". I didn't really believe them, but I wasn't feeling negative. Not believing them provoked and challenged me and I like challenge. By saying "I can't do it" I was building up my impetus to do it and that actually made me feel better. I wasn't trying to delude myself; I knew I had to do it.'*
>
> Gina's use of **integrative power** acts to draw on the integrative power of her environment (**integrated strength**). She does this in a way that only Gina could know would work. And knowing it would work comes from her personal use of **integrative power**.
>
> *'I was in tune with the physicality of the baby. I wasn't in tune with her as a soul. I was very aware of her head coming down my vagina. I needed to reach down and feel her head again; I felt 20 cents worth at my perineum. I couldn't believe I was going to get a head out of there, it felt impossible. I felt stretched to capacity; like I was going to split apart. I made peace with that fear pretty quickly by thinking "oh well, I might not have an intact perineum"... I wasn't really ever fearful, it was more about my confidence... Knowing that I had to do it was what took me from seeing it as impossible to actually doing it.'*
>
> While Gina is experiencing **spiritual territories** she becomes challenged by a sense of impossibility as she accesses **qualified strength** and momentarily experiences the **owned territories**. Yet she uses her **integrative power** again, accesses **integrated strength** and resumes experience of the **spiritual territories** in order to find the new ways of 'being' to actually do it (**genius birth**). She actualizes her potential and gives **genius birth** to her baby using her own power.

To be integrated is powerful. Integration harnesses potential in the here and now of existence and creates possibility. While Emily, Maree, Jane and Gina each used integrative ways of 'being', they also experienced the disconnections of disintegration. Yet it was through the acceptance and courage they gained with integrative ways of 'being', sometimes accessed from their environment, that they were able to change and deflect the disintegration. For Jasmin, on the other hand, disintegrative ways of 'being' dominated to the extent that she could see no other way of 'being'. Each woman's ability to actualize their potential power for birth was therefore influenced by their spiritual practices of enacting integrative ways of 'being'.

CONCLUSION

This chapter has focused on women as 'embodied selves' immersed in the inner and outer environments of ongoing change. It has discussed childbirth change in terms of overall linear change and as intimately ordinary cycles of change. Habitual, institutionalized practices have been identified as socially sanctioned rituals that exclude intimately ordinary change cycles and result in disintegration of 'embodied self'. Rational dichotomous thinking has been recognized as causing and maintaining these disconnective practices. In contrast rituals of familiarity and uniqueness have been shown to be integrative to 'embodied self' by honouring both cyclical and linear childbirth change.

Having illustrated that *non*rational power and knowledge is experientially grounded in 'being', the chapter has shown that ways of 'being' are related to the ever-changing relationship between rational ego boundaries and *non*rational potential. The chapter has argued that we can always choose whether to allow the disconnections of disintegrative ways of 'being' to dominate or to maintain a sense of connected integration through the use of spiritual practices. It has highlighted awareness of *non*rationality as both a possible resource and an outcome of childbirth. In the socio-political arena, the chapter has identified that the *non*rational transformations of natural birth are misinterpreted through rational dichotomous thinking. It has also recognized that this misinterpretation causes the experience of ordinary, intimate change cycles to be ignored and creates difficulties for women and/or midwives intending natural birth.

The chapter has outlined how it is the *way* in which the self changes that most impacts on our ability to actualize our potential. So, as an alternative to the generalized term of natural birth, the chapter has used the theory 'Territories of the Self' to offer the language of ways of 'being', of integration compared with disintegration, and of 'genius birth'. It has illustrated, using women's words, how this language highlights the spiritual practices of moving toward connectivity and integration despite the disconnections of change. The chapter therefore asserts that when spiritual practices are undertaken, the woman is most able to gather her potential, use her power and place herself in the position to experience the best possible, uniquely individual birth appropriate to that particular moment of her life; this is what I call 'genius birth'.

References

Beck C, Driscoll J 2005 Postpartum mood and anxiety disorders. A clinician's guide. Jones and Bartlett, Massachusetts.

Beckett K 2005 Choosing caesarean. Feminism and the politics of childbirth in the United States. Feminist Theory 6(3): 251–275.

Boath E, Pryce A, Cox J 1998 Postnatal depression: The impact on the family. Journal of Reproductive and Infant Psychology 16(2/3): 199–204.

Borders N 2006 After the afterbirth: a critical review of postpartum health relative to method of delivery. Journal of Midwifery and Women's Health 51(4): 242–248.

Brown A 2003 Foucauldian perspectives on midwifery practices and education. Internet Journal of Advanced Nursing Practice 6(1): 15–29.

Brown S, Lumley J 1998 Maternal health after childbirth: results of an Australian population based survey. British Journal of Obstetrics and Gynaecology, 105(2): 156–161.

Chen K 2004 An analytic review of studies on measuring effects of external *qi* in China. Alternative Therapies in Health and Medicine 10(4): 38–50.

Curl J (Ed) 2006 A Dictionary of Architecture and Landscape Architecture. Oxford University Press. Oxford Reference Online. Available: http://0-www.oxfordreference.com. library.newcastle.edu.au:80/views/ENTRY.html? subview=Mainandentry=t1.e5565 10 Oct 2006.

Davis-Floyd R 2003 Birth as an American rite of passage, 2nd edn. University of California Press.

Davis-Floyd R, Davis E 1997 Intuition as authoritative knowledge in midwifery and home birth. In: R Davis-Floyd, P Arvidson (Eds). Intuition: The inside story. University of California Press, Berkeley, pp. 145–176.

DeJudicibus M, McCabe M 2002 Psychological factors and the sexuality of pregnant and postpartum women. Journal of Sex Research 39(2): 94–103.

Downe S, McCourt C 2004 From being to becoming: reconstructing childbirth knowledges. In: S Downe (Ed). Normal childbirth: Evidence and debate. Churchill Livingston, London, pp. 3–24.

Fahy K, Parratt J 2006 Birth territory: A theory for midwifery practice. Women and Birth 19(2): 45–50.

Gaskin I 1990 Spiritual midwifery, 3rd edn. The Book Publishing Company, Tennessee.

Grosz E 1994 Volatile bodies: Toward a corporeal feminism. Allen and Unwin, St Leonards.

Grosz E 1995 Space, time and perversion: The politics of bodies. Allen and Unwin, St Leonards.

Hanh T 1995 Zen Keys: A guide to Zen practice. Doubleday Dell, New York.

Haraway D 2000 A cyborg manifest. In: D Bell, B Kennedy (Eds). The cybercultures reader. Routledge, London, pp. 291–324.

Harcombe J 1999 Power and political power positions in maternity care. British Journal of Midwifery 7(2): 78–82.

Irigaray L 1993 An ethics of sexual difference (Translated by C Burke, G Gill). Athlone, London.

Irigaray L 2001 To be two (Translated by M Monoc, M Rhodes). Routledge, New York.

Johanson R, Wilkinson P, Bastible A et al 1993 Health after childbirth: A comparison of normal and assisted vaginal delivery. Midwifery 9(3): 161–168.

Klassen P 2001 Blessed events: Religion and homebirth in America. Princeton University Press.

Kovel J 1991 History and spirit: An inquiry into the philosophy of liberation. Beacon Press, Boston.

Kristeva J 1982 Powers of horror: An essay on abjection (Translated by L Roudiez). Columbia University Press, New York.

Lacan J 1977 Four fundamental concepts of psycho-analysis (Translated by A Sheridan). Penguin, Harmondsworth.

Lacan J 2004 Écrits: A selection (Translated by B Fink). Norton, London.

Levy V 1999 Midwives, informed choice and power: Part 3. British Journal of Midwifery 7(11): 694–699.

Merleau-Ponty M 2002 The phenomenology of perception. Routledge Classics, London.

Pairman S, Pincombe J, Thorogood C et al (Eds) 2006 Midwifery: Preparation for practice. Elsevier, Sydney.

Parratt J 2005 Stories of the embodied self during childbirth. Self published collection: PO Mandurang Australia 3551.

Parratt J 2008 Feeling like a genius: Women's changing embodied self during childbearing. PhD Thesis, University of Newcastle, Australia.

Parratt J, Fahy K 2003 Trusting enough to be out of control: A pilot study of women's sense of self during childbirth. Australian Journal of Midwifery 16(1): 15–22.

Parratt J, Fahy K 2004 Creating a 'safe' place for birth: An empirically grounded theory. New Zealand College of Midwives Journal 30(1): 11–14.

Parratt J, Fahy K 2008 Including the *non*rational is sensible midwifery. Women and Birth 21(1): 37–42.

Robb C 2006 This changes everything: The relational revolution in psychology. Farrar, Strauss and Giroux, New York.

Roncalli L 1997 Standing by process: A midwife's notes on story-telling, passage, and intuition. In: R Davis-Floyd, P Arvidson (Eds). Intuition: The inside story. University of California Press, Berkeley, pp.177–200.

Sancier K, Holman D 2004 Commentary: Multifaceted Health Benefits of Medical Qigong. Journal of Alternative and Complementary Medicine 10(1): 163–165.

Sterling P 2004 Principles of allostasis. In: J Sckulkin (Ed). Allostasis, homeostasis and the cost of adaption. Cambridge University Press, pp.17–64.

Thompson J, Roberts C, Currie M et al 2002 Prevalence and persistence of health problems after childbirth: Associations with parity and method of birth. Birth 29(2): 83–94.

Trumble W Stevenson A (Eds) 2002 The shorter Oxford English dictionary, 5th edn (Vol 1–2). Oxford University Press.

Turner V 1972 Betwixt and between: The liminal period in rites de passage. In: W Lessa, E Vogt (Eds). Reader in comparative religions: An anthropological approach. Harper and Row, New York.

Tzu L 1963 Tao Te Ching (Translated by D Lau). Penguin Classics, London.

VandeVusse L 1999 Decision making in analyses of women's birth stories. Birth 26(1): 43–50.

van Gennep A 1960 The rites of passage (Translated by M Vizedom, G Caffee). University of Chicago Press.

Vernon D (Ed) 2006 Having a great birth in Australia. Australian College of Midwives, Canberra.

Wilhelm R, Baynes C, (Eds) 1967 The I Ching or Book of changes, 3rd edn. Princeton University Press.

Wynn F 2002 The early relationship of mother and pre-infant: Merleau-Ponty and pregnancy. Nursing Philosophy 3(1): 4–14.

Section 2

Physiology and the physical space

Chapter 5

Creating birth space to enable undisturbed birth

Maralyn Foureur

In 2005 the International Confederation of Midwives (ICM) amended the internationally agreed definition of the midwife to include the italicized words '…care includes …*the promotion of normal birth*' (ICM 2005). These few simple words have legitimized a process that will forever change the rhetoric of 'the midwife is the guardian of normal birth' into reality. However the state of our knowledge of 'normal birth' is so limited by the medically dominated paradigm governing our academic preparation for practice, and how we currently practice, that we will need a new way of thinking about women and birth to bring this about. This chapter will explore three important questions that need to be carefully considered if we are to become true guardians of normal birth:

- What is 'normal birth'?
- Why do we need to promote normal birth?
- How will the future of midwifery education, practice and research be shaped by a new understanding of normal birth?

In order to answer these questions, this chapter focuses on two key areas of scientific knowledge. The first is a relatively new and continuously evolving and expanding understanding of the complex interplay of hormonal influences on childbirth, with an emphasis on the integrative role of the powerful neuro-hormone, Oxytocin. The second is to consider carefully the concepts embraced by the phrase 'nature via nurture', first coined by Matt Ridley in his book of the same name where he explored 'the impact of the environment on our genes' (Ridley 2004). The result of this exploration will be a deeper understanding of how the environment for birth needs to be shaped and protected for normal birth to take place and importantly, how midwives can promote that process by creating birth space that does not disturb healthy physiological processes.

Throughout this chapter I use the capitalized Oxytocin when referring to endogenous, or the woman's naturally produced Oxytocin, whereas when I refer to artificial *oxytocin* I write it without a capital and with italics. This distinction is important to keep in mind. Using evidence from animal and human research with particular emphasis on Oxytocin, this chapter reveals how our interaction with, and feedback from the environment changes the balance between our two predominant bio-behavioural states of 'calm and connection' or 'activation and defence'. Both bio-behavioural states are essential for the maintenance of health and wellbeing. In childbirth the 'calm and connect' state will prevail but this balance can be disrupted if the woman finds herself in unsafe 'birth territory'. The imbalance that results alters the normal neuro-hormonal pathways involved in the birth process. Evidence is provided to illustrate the recent discovery of the role of Oxytocin as not only stimulating uterine contractions and the 'let-down reflex' in breastfeeding, but in a much more complex and expanded role in initiating and maintaining the balance between the two bio-behavioural systems. The chapter continues by exploring how disruptions to the Oxytocin system may be involved in switching on and off components of our individual genetic blueprint as a result of environmental experiences and exposures occurring at any stage of life, but importantly, from (even) the period of pre-conception, throughout the perinatal period and up until we pass through puberty. An awareness of this critical period of 'plasticity' provides us with a strong rationale for guarding the birth space to ensure the prenatal, birth and immediate postnatal environment is optimal for each woman/baby. This knowledge provides midwives with tools to use in creating birth spaces that support women well and thereby provides us with insights into the importance of our role as guardians of the birth space, if we are to ensure that birth remains 'normal'.

A TRANSDISCIPLINARY APPROACH TO THE LITERATURE

I invite you take a journey with me as I traverse a wide array of literature drawn from many scientific and humanistic disciplines; from research published often decades ago to that published currently, and through a range of research conducted across species as disparate as rodents, sheep, non-human primates and humans. This journey requires that you accept the premise that there are fundamental physiological processes in play during pregnancy and parturition and immediately after birth that are similar across all mammalian species and across time (Naaktgeboren 1989; Odent 1999). Integration of knowledge from across multiple sources, however, needs to be undertaken with caution. Extrapolating from animal research and behaviour to human behaviour and physiology is a somewhat risky activity since we assume that humans are less governed by 'basic instinctual behaviour' and more able to be influenced by society, culture, morality and ethical choices in behaviour. In this chapter I will highlight any areas where particular caution needs to be exercised when extrapolating from animals to humans.

As well as being 'cross disciplinary' and 'cross species', the research was conducted in a variety of ways and includes empirical research, true experiments, randomized controlled trials, cohort and longitudinal studies, case–control studies, observational and qualitative research. All have a contribution to make to the understanding of the complex nature of the impact of the environment on birth. What we are seeking is to identify patterns in these disparate fields of inquiry that will help us to better understand normal birth and how to keep birth normal. There are patterns emerging in discoveries from many scientific fields that contribute small pieces of greater understanding to this complex puzzle. Much of this knowledge is still at the stage of hypothesis generating research and theory development. These theories will provide the stimulus for much future research since the discovery and mapping of the human genome has enabled new and exciting insights into our very being and what makes us who we individually are.

CONTINUITY OF MIDWIFERY CARE

I began my own search for pieces of the physiology of normal birth puzzle over 10 years ago with a randomized controlled trial (RCT) of continuity of midwifery care (Rowley et al 1995). I am passionately interested in discovering ways to support women during childbirth to ensure that they have a positive experience. My focus is to support women in ways that prevent unnecessary obstetric intervention because it is apparent that any intervention often has serious consequences of its own. From my practice as a self-employed midwife from the early 1980s onwards, I had discovered that getting to know women during pregnancy and being able to provide them with one-to-one care throughout labour and the birth of the baby, resulted in hardly any fetal distress or slow labour necessitating obstetric intervention. I wanted every woman having a baby to be able to receive one-to-one care because I had a hunch that this support made a difference to the birth process and therefore the outcome. However, women who accessed this kind of care were clearly a particular subsection of the community, namely, mostly older, middle class, white, English speakers and non smokers who were highly motivated to seek midwifery led maternity care and strive for a normal birth. I wondered whether it might simply be the characteristics and motivation of the women that led to their high rates of birth without any obstetric intervention. In order to test whether my hunch was right and to persuade the maternity community that this was a safe model of care that all women should have access to, it was apparent that I would need to be able to provide answers to two important questions: is this kind of care effective and is it what women want? Only a randomized controlled trial could answer these questions.

DEVELOPING THEORY: THE FEAR CASCADE IN LABOUR

The RCT of continuity of midwifery care was conducted with a small team of midwives (Rowley et al 1995). It did provide strong evidence of both effectiveness and women's satisfaction with continuity of midwifery care (as have many other studies since 1995). During the research period I developed a theory as to why one-to-one care might make such a difference. I read an inspiring paper by a team of researchers (Sosa et al 1980) describing an RCT which they conducted in Guatemala where they also revealed that women provided with 'a supportive companion', had fewer interventions in childbirth and healthier babies (higher Apgar scores, fewer admissions to neonatal intensive care). In this setting women usually laboured alone, with no-one in constant attendance. The study had provided each woman with the support of a doula; an 'untrained' birth companion. The authors also pondered what mechanism could be operating to influence such outcomes. They hypothesized that being alone in labour meant that women became anxious and fearful; an emotional state in which the autonomic nervous system may take over many physiological functions by releasing a range of substances in the brain (for a more detailed understanding of the autonomic nervous system see Uvnäs-Moberg 2003). Sosa and his colleagues were particularly interested in the role of adrenaline which was known to inhibit the release of Oxytocin that is required to make the uterus contract and labour to progress. I examined this hypothesis carefully by pouring over the physiology texts until I thought I understood the mechanism well and ultimately produced a plausible theoretical explanation which I called the Fear Cascade, illustrated in Figure 5.1 (Rowley 1998; Foureur 2005; Foureur and Hunter 2006).

The Fear Cascade acknowledges that once labour has begun, there are two main reasons for all intervention in childbirth. These are, uterine inertia and fetal distress (ill-defined constructs though they may be). The theory explains why

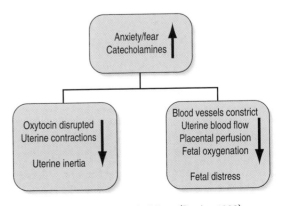

Figure 5.1 The fear cascade in labour (Rowley 1998).

this is so by suggesting that if women become acutely stressed (psychologically or physiologically) during labour, the nervous system will automatically (and unconsciously) respond by initiating the well known 'fight-or-flight' reaction described by Walter Cannon in 1932 and well researched since then (Taylor et al 2000). Flooding the brain and every body system with the stress hormones, cortisol, vasopressin and the catecholamines; adrenaline and nor-adrenaline, impacts the body's physiological (and mental) processes. In labour, adrenaline has the ability to disrupt the rhythmical release of endogenous Oxytocin, and may slow it down or block secretion entirely (Shnider and Levinson 1987). Labour will normally become either irregular, slow down or stop (Hutton 1986; Simkin 1986; Simkin and Ancheta 2000). Midwives know this process well and it is now accepted that when labouring women are first admitted to hospital, labour may slow until they 'settle in' when it will naturally resume. This understanding provides part of the rationale for having women bring support people with them, or for guided tours of the labour room during pregnancy so that women may become more familiar with the environment for birth and are less fearful. In some instances, nor-adrenaline will be the more powerful hormone triggered by the nervous system. Nor-adrenaline has the opposite effect to adrenaline; dramatically increasing the release of Oxytocin thereby initiating the 'precipitous labour' (or fetal ejection reflex) seen in some women, and another process very familiar to midwives. All of us have stories of women who appeared to meet some crisis point in labour where cervical dilatation moved from 1–2 cm to the birth of the baby in a matter of seconds or minutes.

The Fear Cascade also demonstrates a plausible explanation for fetal distress as a consequence of acute maternal stress during labour. The release of adrenaline will not only disrupt release of Oxytocin, but also has an effect on the walls of blood vessels, narrowing those supplying what the body considers to be 'non-essential' organs during a situation of 'fight-or-flight'. Blood is diverted to the brain (for clear thinking) and to the muscles (to run away from danger or face a foe and be able to fight). The Fear Cascade hypothesizes that the fear-adrenaline initiated process will constrict blood vessels supplying the uterus since it is considered a non-essential organ during a fearful situation. Even a small reduction in the volume of blood supplied to the uterus and subsequently the placenta, will cause fetal distress to soon become apparent (Shnider et al 1987; Nathanielsz 1992; Mead 1996; Mongan 2005).

EVIDENCE IN SUPPORT OF THE FEAR CASCADE

In my search for evidence to support my developing theory I turned to biology and began considering evidence from animal experiments.

Environmental stress induces uterine inertia

The work of a perinatal psychologist, Niles Newton has been foundational to understanding the impact of the perinatal environment on birthing (Newton et al 1966a, 1966b, 1968; Newton 1986, 1990). Newton published a large number of studies from the 1960s up to the 1990s. These studies focused on the consequences of perinatal environmental disturbance which she investigated through research conducted on a variety of small mammals including laboratory mice and rats. In a series of carefully designed experiments with mice, Newton explored the impact of giving birth in a hostile environment and I will describe several of the experiments here.

Newton began her investigations by rotating pregnant mice at term, between a glass bowl containing bedding contaminated with cat urine (a hostile and stress filled environment) and their usual darkened nesting box (a safe space). Significantly fewer mice delivered their babies in the hostile environment. The next experiment concentrated on timing the length of labour when one group of mice was disturbed by handling and a comparison group was left undisturbed. Again a significant difference was found with the disturbed mice exhibiting labours of up to 65–72% longer. A third experiment saw one group of mice rotated between two hostile locations and another between two familiar locations. The results showed that the mice in the hostile environments delivered their pups 4–3 hours later than controls. Unexpectedly, the total time from the delivery of the first of the litter to the last was much shorter for the mice in the hostile environment. This suggested an initial slowing of labour followed by precipitous delivery. Newton proposed therefore that slowing labour while seeking a safe environment for the birth appears to be a normal adaptive response. However, once the baby is in the birth canal it is not as easy for the mother to move, hence there is a survival advantage to rapidly emptying the birth canal. Of considerable concern was the finding on the day following birth that the pups of the groups that were continuously disturbed or who were born in the hostile location were more likely to be found dead than mice born in the familiar and safe environment. This suggests some form of fetal damage occurred during labour or birth in the hostile environment.

Newton wondered:

> '... are mammals with more highly developed nervous systems than the mouse equally sensitive to perinatal environmental disturbance...what effect if any does variation [between home and hospital environments] have on the course of labor and infant mortality?' (Newton 1972, p. 13)

Further evidence in support of the Fear Cascade emerged from studies in nonhuman primates whose behaviour is considered to be more similar to that of humans.

Stress hormone induces fetal asphyxia

In a study by Adamsons et al (1971) fetal asphyxia and acidosis were induced by injecting a catecholamine (adrenaline in this case) into a pregnant rhesus monkey. In an earlier experiment when adrenaline had been injected directly into her fetus through the mother's abdomen, the adrenaline had little effect other than to speed up the heart rate of the fetus. The researchers subsequently found they were able to induce fetal asphyxia and acidosis when the adrenaline was injected into the mother. The researchers postulated that the fetal asphyxia was the result of the vasoconstrictor effect of the adrenaline on the maternal circulation, leading to restricted uterine blood flow and ultimately impacting on placental blood flow and thereby blood flow to the fetal monkey.

In a more recent study with 100 pregnant women (mean gestation 32 weeks) and using colour Doppler ultrasound, researchers demonstrated similar findings in humans (Teixeira et al 1999). Maternal anxiety, measured using standard psychology tools (Spielberger state and trait anxiety), was found to be strongly associated with increased uterine artery resistance index. Increased resistance to blood flow through the uterine artery reduces blood flow to the fetus. The researchers postulated that maternal anxiety therefore appears to affect fetal development and wellbeing and may be implicated in the initiation of premature birth. Increased uterine artery resistance is also associated with babies who are small for gestational age, thus indicating a disruption to normal placental perfusion and nourishment of the fetus.

At this point in my journey to understanding I felt I had discovered ample confirmation of the theoretical model of the Fear Cascade. What I read confirmed for me that continuous, one-to-one support in labour from a midwife known to the woman, would prevent fear from escalating to the point where adrenaline production was stimulated to the level that impaired both uterine contractions and fetal oxygenation. I postulated that continuous one-to-one labour support from a known midwife would help the woman to feel safe and thereby prevent disruption to the Oxytocin secretion process with the consequence that normal labour would occur and fetal distress would be prevented.

I now know that this was a reasonable but somewhat simplistic view of the dynamic interplay of hormones, emotions and childbirth labour. Catecholamines and Oxytocin have even more complex roles to play and of course there are many other hormones involved, although Oxytocin remains the major orchestrator and integrator of neuro-hormonal activity. Part of the reason my initial understanding was limited was the inadequacy of previous ways of researching and explaining how stress operates in humans. New scientific discoveries have now made it possible to understand much more about what is likely to be happening.

GENDER BIAS IN STRESS STUDIES

The first area to be challenged is that when women are stressed and frightened they automatically experience a 'fight-or-flight' response. We now understand that contemporary text books may be based on an outdated and incorrect understanding of how stress operates in women's bodies. Most of the research that has increased our understanding of this catecholamine mediated, automatic process, was conducted with young, white, males (Taylor et al 2000). Males became the subjects of choice since the results of experiments with women were inconsistent, sometimes inconclusive or outcomes tended in the opposite direction. The normal cyclical variation in neuro-endocrine function that women experience throughout the menstrual cycle was postulated as the explanation for these contradictory findings. Researchers simply stopped exploring the physiology of the 'fight-or-flight' response in women. An assumption was made that since this was a basic physiological process, it would be identical no matter what gender. Researchers now consider this assumption may be wrong.

BALANCING SYSTEMS: FIGHT–OR–FLIGHT AND CALM AND CONNECTION

New research has revealed the 'fight-or-flight' response is not the first automatic response to stress in women that it appears to be in most (but not all) men (Geary and Flynn 2002). There is an equally powerful stress response at work in women that has the opposite reaction to what occurs for men. It has been termed the 'calm and connection' response (or 'tend-and-befriend' response) and it appears to have evolved to provide women with an ability to react to stressful situations in an energy conserving way (Taylor et al 2000; Uvnäs-Moberg 2003). Some of the opposing components of these two systems are demonstrated in Table 5.1.

Theory of the balancing systems: the role of Oxytocin

Researchers working in different areas of scientific inquiry have developed a theoretical understanding of why the stress reactions of men and women may differ and this is what they propose (Taylor et al 2000). The 'fight-or-flight' response is an important survival mechanism for both men and women but possibly more so for the male of the species since phylogenetically speaking, males who were once meat hunters, are built for speed, to run away from predators and for defence of territory and 'breeding space'. This behaviour is mediated by the hormone testosterone. However for women, who have the responsibility of babies and young children or who might be pregnant, running from a potential threat may not be possible. Therefore an additional mechanism has developed that enables women (and their dependent children) to survive. Put simply it involves a process of seeking affiliative relationships; linking and bonding with others and calming behaviours in the face of threat (Taylor et al 2000). This response is facilitated by Oxytocin and endogenous opioid mechanisms. One proposal is that this response to stress/threat/fear may be the female adult counterpart of the infant attachment mechanism which we know is crucial for '...normal biological regulatory systems in offspring' (Taylor et al 2000, p. 412). This response has been called the tend-and-befriend system by one research group (Taylor et al 2000) or the calm-and-connection system by others

Table 5.1   Key features of the two bio-behavioural states

Calm and connection	Fight–or–flight
Mentally calm, alert and open to communication and interaction	Mentally hyper-alert and aggressive/defensive or
Improved learning	Mentally frozen
Lowered heart rate	Increased heart rate
Lowered blood pressure	Elevated blood pressure
Increased circulation to the skin	Increased blood to muscles
Increased sensitivity to touch	Insensitivity of skin
Inhibition of release of glucocorticoids	Extra fuel from release of glucose from liver
More effective digestion, nutritional uptake and storage	Decreased activity of digestive system
Higher pain threshold (increased tolerance for pain)	
Lower levels of stress hormones	Higher level of stress hormones
High levels of Oxytocin	High levels of adrenaline, noradrenaline and cortisol
Mediated by oestrogen	Mediated by testosterone

(Carter 2003; Uvnäs-Moberg 2003). In the rest of the chapter it will be referred to as the calm-and-connection system.

OXYTOCIN MEDIATES PHYSIOLOGY AND BEHAVIOUR

This new understanding of the female response to stress has been made possible by recent discoveries concerning the major role that the neuro-hormone Oxytocin plays in mediating a vast range of mindbody processes. While Oxytocin is present in both males and females it is potentiated by oestrogen, therefore has its most clearly demonstrated effects on females, in particular pregnant and lactating women (Uvnäs-Moberg 2003). Oxytocin is the key to the calm-and-connection system. Oxytocin is involved in much more than the mechanical aspects of labour, childbirth and breastfeeding. We are just beginning to discover how important it is and why protecting and promoting normal birth is essential for our survival as a species (Carter 2003; Carter et al 1995).

Since Oxytocin is a neuro-hormone, it is secreted in the brain as well as in different sites in the body. As a neuro-hormone it acts centrally as well as locally which means that Oxytocin influences behaviour as well as having a localized impact on different body systems. The localized mechanical impact of Oxytocin on the uterus and breasts are the processes with which midwives are most familiar. In the brain Oxytocin is a neurotransmitter, linking messages throughout the vast network of nerves in the brain and spinal column and therefore influences many body systems and behaviours, but particularly behaviours that are characteristic of the calm-and-connection system. In shorthand terms, Oxytocin initiates love.

Oxytocin initiates love

Niles Newton was the first researcher to formally make the observation that Oxytocin could appropriately be called the love hormone since it was always associated with affiliative behaviours such as pair bonding in animals; the attachment and nesting behaviour seen between mothers and their babies, and it was always present during sexual activities. This behavioural role for Oxytocin has been confirmed by many studies in both animals and humans and I will explore some of those here.

Oxytocin is a challenging hormone on which to conduct research because it does not cross the 'blood–brain barrier'. What we can measure in the blood taken from venepuncture in the peripheries of the body (arms or legs) may not be reflective of levels in the brain (Carter 2003; Uvnäs-Moberg 2003). Here is a word of caution. While correlations between levels of Oxytocin in the blood and cerebrospinal-fluid (CSF) have been demonstrated and correlations between either CSF or blood levels of Oxytocin and behaviour exist, evidence of Oxytocin produced in the brain and subsequent behavioural changes, in humans, is still indirect. If we want to understand the behavioural effects of the hormone then we need to be able to measure the levels of Oxytocin that are present in the brain in direct relation to a particular behaviour. Therefore most of the research into the behavioural consequences of Oxytocin has been performed with animals. Using ethical research processes, the brains of experimental animals have been cannulated so that levels of Oxytocin can be directly measured and manipulated.

OXYTOCIN RESEARCH WITH ANIMALS

In the following section I explore Oxytocin research with three mammals; the prairie vole, sheep and non-human primates to illustrate some of the behavioural effects of this and other hormones during the perinatal period.

The prairie vole

Prairie voles are highly social, monogamous rodents found in mid-western North America. They mate for life and such is the strength of their pair bond, male and female travel their habitat in constant touch with each other; side by side, sharing the nesting and caretaking of their offspring. Researchers have discovered that the brain of the prairie vole is awash with Oxytocin (especially when compared with their antisocial cousins the montane voles) making them ideal subjects for research that manipulates Oxytocin levels and measures subsequent changes in affiliative and parenting behaviour (Williams et al 1994; Angier 1999; Cushing and Carter 2000; Carter 2003).

Oxytocin production in the brain can be blocked by injecting an Oxytocin antagonist (e.g. Atosiban) directly into the brain. Dramatic behavior change results when an Oxytocin antagonist is injected into the brain of a female prairie vole. The female stops taking care of her pups and exhibiting nesting behaviour, and rejects her mate, becoming hostile towards any physical contact. When the Oxytocin antagonist is removed, the female starts nesting again and becomes re-attached to her mate (Carter 2003). This is strong evidence in support of Oxytocin as the hormone of love and attachment, at least in animals.

Further research has demonstrated that Oxytocin is not only involved in sexual activity; male and female orgasm; labour contractions; fetal ejection reflex at birth; placental ejection reflex and breastfeeding, but it is also stimulated by touch and rhythmical stroking and is a key participant in eating behaviour (Verbalis et al 1986; Gimpl et al 2001; Uvnäs-Moberg 2003). We will encounter the prairie vole again later in the chapter.

The ewe and the lamb

Research in parturient sheep has long been of interest to perinatologists and other scientists since much of pregnant ewe and lamb physiology and behaviour, parallels that of parturient women (Da Costa et al 1996). Sheep farmers are also very familiar with the importance of attachment and bonding behaviour during lambing to ensure the survival of the flock. Their knowledge is also useful for perinatal researchers interested in understanding more about human birth.

We know that sheep 'bond like glue' within one hour of birth and if the mother and her lamb are separated at this crucial time, they will never bond. A lamb who is not bonded to its mother will be rejected when it attempts to feed and will ultimately not survive. However, researchers have discovered that *oxytocin* injected directly into the brain of the ewe will result in the ewe bonding instantly with any lamb it is shown (Kendrick et al 1987). Oxytocin facilitates a mechanism whereby the mother rapidly learns to recognize which is her baby. We now understand that this Oxytocin mediated process may be triggered by smell (Curtis et al 2001). Through careful observation of sheep behaviour, farmers have known this for some time. For example, occasionally either a ewe or lamb will die during childbirth. If a ewe's lamb dies and another lamb needs a

mother, the farmer will place the skin of the dead lamb on the motherless lamb and it will be accepted by the ewe. The ewe has recognized the foster lamb as her own by its smell.

The role of smell in attachment behaviour has been confirmed by other studies. One group of researchers has noticed that animals (in this case, rats) who are housed in the same cage with research animals who have been injected with *exogenous oxytocin* exhibit the same Oxytocin related calm and connection behaviours as if they had received the *oxytocin* injection too, although to a lesser extent (Uvnäs-Moberg 2003). When the ability to smell is blocked temporarily in the cage-mates, the calm and connection behaviours disappear.

In other behavioural research with sheep, studies have established that there is also a link between the gut and the brain. Suckling releases Oxytocin in the lamb's brain and simultaneously cholescystokinin in the lamb's gut. If either Oxytocin or cholescystokinin are blocked (by injecting Oxytocin or cholescystokinin antagonists into the lamb), the ability of the lamb to bond with its mother is disrupted.

Other researchers have established that epiduralized sheep or those who give birth by caesarean section will not bond with their lamb after birth (Krehbiel et al 1987). In subsequent studies, researchers have stimulated Oxytocin release and bonding in these instances by inserting a device (dildo) into the ewe's vagina to stretch it, with the result that the ewe will again bond instantly with any lamb it is shown (Angier 1999). The stretching of the vaginal wall simulates the passage of the lamb through the birth canal, thereby stimulating the Ferguson reflex which also appears to be a critical component of the Oxytocin attachment process (Segal 2001, 2002; El-Hamamy and Arulkumaran 2005).

These are just a few of the thought provoking examples of Oxytocin and the calm and connection system at work in sheep. Now we will turn to similar studies in non human primates whose physiology and attachment behaviour mirrors that of humans even more closely.

The Bonobo

The Bonobo (or pygmy ape), a close African relative of humans is a unique mammal. The

Bonobo have much to teach us about the potential role of Oxytocin in influencing behaviour at a group or societal level. The Bonobo are highly social creatures who live in a female-centred (possibly even female-dominated), peace-loving and egalitarian society that substitutes Oxytocin inducing sexual acts for aggression (de Waal 1995) and their brains are flooded with Oxytocin. Many forms of sexual activity (grooming, hugging, kissing, touching, genital rubbing, intercourse – both heterosexual and homosexual) are a casual and relatively common (although not continuous) feature of the social life of the Bonobo. Oxytocin infused public displays of affection and sexual acts are used to maintain harmony by defusing stress and aggression in all forms; competition for food, for space, for partners; to make up after an argument; to appease and to bond with other members of the group. Sex is not used to achieve climactic release but as the major form of communication and relationship building.

Males and females are less aggressive and hot tempered than their chimpanzee cousins and are much less likely to resort to physical violence in any form. By using sexual overtures female Bonobos form close social bonds with unrelated females that establish their status in Bonobo society. Males derive their status and protection from their mothers. Unlike most other non-human primates, the male Bonobo actively participates in parental behaviour. Researchers suggest that the Bonobo is the prototypical human ancestor and their behaviour demonstrates what human society would look like if we had evolved in the same way, without hierarchies and male dominance maintained by aggression (Angier 1997). Such is the power of Oxytocin to positively influence calm and connection behaviours in an entire society.

Interestingly men who exhibit high levels of caring parental behaviour and who do not automatically respond to stress with the fight-or-flight response (like Bonobo males) were found in one study to have low levels of testosterone and high levels of prolactin (Geary et al 2002). Prolactin and Oxytocin have '...a variety of interactions and may act as releasing factors for each other...[thus], the presence or absence of prolactin might have indirect effects on Oxytocin and vice

versa' (Carter 2003, p. 393). In the study of high parental men, testosterone/prolactin hormonal patterns were highly correlated with, and therefore probably influenced by, the nature of the man's relationship with his wife (Geary et al 2002). The stronger the bond between the two, the higher the prolactin level and the lower the testosterone. The literature does not report the testosterone/prolactin pattern in Bonobo males but parallels may exist.

OXYTOCIN RESEARCH IN CHILDBEARING AND LACTATING WOMEN

In her recently published book *The Oxytocin Factor*, physiologist Kerstin Uvnäs-Moberg (2003) outlines the major discoveries in the area of Oxytocin research from her unit in the Karolinska Institute in Sweden. With the assistance of midwives she has been exploring the nature of Oxytocin in pregnant and lactating women and their babies for many years. In these studies Oxytocin levels are measured in blood obtained from a cannula in the mother's arm. Blood is extracted at one minute intervals for periods of up to 10 minutes during pregnancy, labour and birth or breastfeeding, enabling the identification of the pulsatile release of Oxytocin and the discovery that each woman has an individual pattern of Oxytocin release. A range of physiological and behavioural measurements and observations are made of the mothers and their interactions with their infants allowing the team to identify that in mothers Oxytocin is anxiolytic (i.e. reduces or prevents anxiety) and analgesic (increases the threshold for pain); facilitates learning, attachment and parenting behaviour. The major finding is that Oxytocin orchestrates a process of energy conservation throughout the mother's body in order for her to have sufficient ability to grow a new human in utero, then to be able to ensure its survival by producing sufficient nutrients in breastmilk, without threatening her own survival.

The feelings associated with centrally released Oxytocin are calmness and a desire to increase social interaction with others. Uvnäs-Moberg focuses on lactating women because we are aware that during this period, women's bodies are flooded with Oxytocin and we can reasonably infer from the animal studies previously examined that what can be measured peripherally in blood plasma is reflective of levels occurring in the brain. The research team has discovered that following the birth of their baby, breastfeeding women are more social and less anxious than non breastfeeding women. These personality changes persist for up to six months after the birth and the onset of the personality change is more rapid in multiparous women. The research also reveals that the higher the level of Oxytocin, the more calm and social the mother. Thereby, stress is reduced; levels of the stress hormone cortisol drop; pain threshold is increased (through integration of the endorphin system); body temperature is regulated (increasing temperature of the breasts) and heart rate and blood pressure are also lowered. Interestingly blood pressure is lowered in breastfeeding women in both the short and long-term with the long-term changes dependent on, and proportionately reflecting, the length of time spent breastfeeding. The long-term effect cannot be directly attributed to Oxytocin since it disappears from the blood rapidly. Instead it is apparent that Oxytocin must influence, or 'switch on' some other process in a long standing way. The ability of Oxytocin to switch on other processes will be returned to later in this chapter.

Uvnäs-Moberg states that the net result of the calming influence of Oxytocin is that maternal energy is conserved; energy that is required to meet the caloric requirements of producing nutrients for the baby. The sleepiness many women report when breastfeeding is another sign of Oxytocin acting centrally to conserve energy by changing maternal behaviour. Breast feeding women experience a sense of calm and a desire for seclusion and less interest in stimulation from their environment.

The team at the Karolinksa has also discovered that Oxytocin works to improve the mother's learning abilities, enhances her social memory (for faces) and facilitates affiliative behaviours such as love, altruism and attachment (Uvnäs-Moberg 1997). Oxytocin can be induced by certain smells only able to be detected by very primitive parts of the olfactory system; Oxytocin can be induced in social situations; by tone of voice; by a pleasant approach; by suggesting caring and comfort; by imagining pleasant situations; when having a meal with friends or family around a table (see discussion of cholecystokinin above) and importantly through touch, such as hugging, cuddling, stroking, massage and grooming behaviour (e.g. touching the face when washing, brushing the hair etc).

Touch and Oxytocin

We can sense the world as threatening or pleasant through our skin. Sensations of warmth, cold, light or heavy touch and pain, either stimulate or inhibit the Oxytocin system. Pleasant touch delivered at the rate of 40 beats per minute appears to be the most effective at initiating the calm and connection system (Uvnäs-Moberg 2003). When the baby is placed in skin to skin contact with his mother, he moves his hands to massage the mother's breasts resulting in spikes of Oxytocin in the mother (Uvnäs-Moberg 2004). During breastfeeding, the stimulation of Oxytocin in turn initiates vasodilation of the skin of the mother's chest and abdomen; thus warmth is generated. The baby becomes calm while feeding and the mother also feels calm and sleepy. But there are even more beneficial effects for the mother. Uvnäs-Moberg reports that mothers who experience skin to skin contact with their infants in the first few hours of life not only breastfeed for longer but also have more milk; lower gastrin levels four days later and have a more pulsatile pattern of Oxytocin release with increased sociability related to the number of pulses of Oxytocin. The mothers also react with lower levels of cortisol to stressful events.

Many of the physiological responses seen in the breastfeeding mother are also stimulated by massage (Uvnas-Moberg 2004). Experiments using animals such as rats treated with massage-like stroking have demonstrated all of the effects described above. Since an Oxytocin antagonist injected into the rat counteracted these effects we can reasonably assume that Oxytocin is the initiator and integrator of these responses. An interesting application of this knowledge can be seen in the report of a German dairy farmer who developed a 'body brush' for his cows similar to a car wash. The body brush delivered strokes to the sides and backs of the cows resulting in more relaxed animals that produced 26% more milk (Uvnäs-Moberg 2003). In one human study, researchers demonstrated increases in Oxytocin secretion in the massage therapist, as well as the recipients of the massage, indicating that the effect may be bidirectional.

We now know that mothers secrete Oxytocin when they stroke their babies, slowly and rhythmically; animals lick their babies at the rate of 40 beats per minute – the rhythm inducing Oxytocin release. Warm water has the same Oxytocin-inducing effect. Touch that activates Oxytocin production, which in turn enhances nutrient absorption, is one of the underlying principles of 'kangaroo care' for preterm neonates where increased rates of growth were observed following periods of skin-to-skin contact. The oral stimulation of non-nutritive sucking also initiates Oxytocin release and has a calming effect on babies.

Increased understanding about the sense of touch and Oxytocin is a small part of emerging knowledge. New research is making it increasingly apparent that all our sense modalities (sight, hearing, smell, touch and taste) provide input into the Oxytocin system and therefore play an integral role in the bio-behavioural regulation of childbirth.

DISRUPTING THE OXYTOCIN SYSTEM

During childbirth there are many ways in which the normal Oxytocin mediated calm and connection system can be disrupted. Epidural anaesthesia/analgesia for pain relief, birth by caesarean section, artificial feeding of the infant, and inducing or augmenting labour with artificial oxytocin will be briefly considered.

Epidural and caesarean section

In one study women who received an epidural during childbirth reported higher levels of pain the following day when compared with mothers who did not have an epidural. Uvnäs-Moberg (2003) suggests this may be because blocking the release of endogenous Oxytocin which is a consequence of the epidural also interferes with synthesis of Oxytocin which takes some time after the removal of the epidural to recommence. Oxytocin is involved in the initiation and integration of the endorphin response to pain. What effect this disruption to the endogenous Oxytocin system

has on other Oxytocin mediated behaviours we do not know.

We have already seen in studies with epiduralized sheep or those who give birth by caesarean, that the Ferguson reflex is an integral part of the Oxytocin-mediated attachment process. Failure to initiate the Ferguson reflex by feeling the baby pass through the vagina resulted in the ewe failing to recognize its lamb. The same result cannot be directly inferred for women who are epiduralized or give birth by caesarean since it is possible to imagine love and attachment and we are socially conditioned to do so. However there are many accounts of women post caesarean who have reported feeling detached from their infants and wondering if they are truly their own baby. Some accounts can be found on websites such as Birthrites (www.birthrights.com). One study has revealed that caesarean section influences the subsequent pulsatile release of Oxytocin (disrupting the rhythm or decreasing the number of pulses) as well as inhibiting maternal responses to the infant (Nissen et al 1998).

Artificial feeding

Oxytocin occurs naturally in human breast milk as well as being released in the infant itself through suckling and the tactile stimulation received from its mother. Therefore bottle feeding is not simply a matter of replacing one form of nutrients with another. Babies who are bottle fed may also receive less Oxytocin because they receive less tactile stimulation in two ways; less holding by their mother during feeding and less suckling induced release of Oxytocin. In studies using animal models and the presence or absence of the Oxytocin related hormone, prolactin in maternal milk, consequences such as diminished brain growth, altered reactions to stress in later life (hyperresponsiveness), and various forms of reproductive dysfunction including non-ovulatory, polycystic ovaries have been identified (Carter 2003). This suggests the presence of particular hormones in human breastmilk together with the tactile stimulation of the infant through suckling and touching by its mother during breastfeeding may also influence and alter the entire Oxytocin system neuro-anatomy and physiology and hence behaviour. This is yet another example of the role of Oxytocin in switching on or off other processes within the body with lifelong implications.

Artificial oxytocin

Carol Sue Carter, Professor of Psychiatry at the University of Illinois, Chicago, has spent many years studying the neurobiology of social monogamy in prairie voles. Her long-term goal is to develop what she calls 'translational animal models' for understanding the impact of the perinatal environment on our genes and subsequent behaviour. Carter considers the environment to be both the social and hormonal perinatal experiences to which the developing and newly born infant is exposed. Her particular focus is on the way responses to stress can be permanently altered or upregulated by an anxiety filled perinatal environment, potentially leading to behavioural disturbances such as autism. Examples of her research have already been cited in this chapter, but one further aspect of her work needs to be considered in relation to the strengthening of the rationale for keeping birth normal. In a recent paper, Carter articulates an idea that has been considered by other researchers and clinicians; that is, the possible teratogenic (gene damaging) hazards of maternal *exogenous (or artificial) oxytocin* infusion for the fetus (Carter 2003).

Most studies of the impact of *exogenous oxytocin* infusion have only considered the immediate short-term impact on expediting the birth of the baby. None have adequately considered potentially serious, long-term impacts on the fetus and the epigenetic changes that might be initiated. Two aspects of endogenous Oxytocin and *exogenous oxytocin* need to be considered. Firstly, a normal rise in endogenous Oxytocin can be expected as labour progresses to the birth of the baby. Any procedure such as an elective caesarean section that prevents the occurrence of this normal progression in the release of Oxytocin (which in turn interacts with a number of other hormones) may have serious maladaptive consequences. On the other hand, a long and complicated labour which elongates the period during which endogenous Oxytocin is secreted may similarly disrupt a normal process, exposing the body and brain of the infant to abnormally high levels. Either situation may have long-term consequences. Finally the assumption

that *exogenous oxytocin* administered to the mother does not cross the placental barrier in amounts sufficient to influence the fetus may also be found to be false. Carter suggests that the permeability of the maternal–fetal barrier may fluctuate during labour and birth which is the very time when clinicians are likely to administer large amounts of *exogenous oxytocin*. Carter warns '... the small but growing literature in animals suggests .... the assumption that perinatal [Oxytocin/*oxytocin*] manipulations are without effect... may be an invalid assumption' (Carter 2003, p. 392).

Uvnäs-Moberg and her team have discovered that mothers who receive an epidural during childbirth are less calm and less close to their baby (at least for one day after birth). In addition they have reported that large amounts of *artificial oxytocin* to induce or augment labour (which is usually a consequence of an epidural) stimulates the production of vasopressin which has an antidiuretic effect resulting in fluid retention; the risk of post partum haemorrhage increases; breastfeeding is impaired and in the long term, suppresses the production of endogenous Oxytocin.

INFLUENCE OF ENVIRONMENT/ EXPERIENCE ON OUR GENES

There are many patterns of behaviour becoming apparent as a consequence of research into Oxytocin. There have been several large population based cohort studies that have identified behavioural correlations with events which can be described as malfunctions of the Oxytocin system (Odent 1999). These apparent consequences include the serious mental health issues of schizophrenia, autism, drug dependency, suicidal tendencies, antisocial and criminal behaviour, as well as cardiovascular disease (Carter 2003). These can all be conceptualized as signs of an inability to love oneself or others and are all possibly linked to disruptions to the normal Oxytocin-induced behaviours during the critical period surrounding pregnancy, childbirth and breastfeeding.

Oxytocin (and other steroid hormones such as oestrogen that can influence the Oxytocin system) has been found to influence cell growth and death and is therefore implicated in the later appearance of some cancers. Oxytocin neurons in some animal models have been found to have an 'exceptional capacity to change shape and form new synapses'. Oxytocin producing cells can be influenced by Oxytocin themselves and are particularly sensitive to exogenous or artificial sources of *oxytocin* (Carter 2003).

Some confirmation of these links emerged recently in the form of descriptions of the complex interplay between genes and life experiences. One longitudinal study started in Dunedin, New Zealand in the 1970s, has followed a cohort of around 1000 individuals for 32 years. This study has identified a link between the COMT Gene and cannabis use in adolescence. COMT (Catechol O-methyltransferase) is required for the metabolic breakdown of dopamine, a neurotransmitter hypothesized to influence human cognitive function (Malhotra et al 2002). Using cannabis by the age of 15 results in a four times higher risk of adult psychosis or schizophrenia-like disorder through switching off this gene (OR 4.50, 95% CI 1.11–18.21) (Arseneault et al 2002). What this landmark study confirms is that the genetic blueprint is plastic until adolescence and environmental exposures to any number of experiences or events during early life can switch on and off different parts of the genetic blueprint. In this case an opiate-type drug (cannabis) has interacted with a particular gene to significantly alter cognitive functioning resulting in mental illness. Since Oxytocin is the main integrator of neurotransmitters, metabolic functions and behavioural states, it is implicated in this process although exactly how is yet to be identified. This opens the way for further research that may more clearly establish the links between perinatal exposure to a range of artificial or naturally occurring neuro-transmitters (such as Oxytocin) and subsequent switching on or off of genes thereby altering cognitive functioning.

The Barker hypothesis is yet another confirmation that pre and perinatal exposure to environmental challenges may switch on or off parts of each individual's genetic blueprint resulting in a wide range of physical, physiological and behavioural consequences that are intergenerational (Barker 1998; Barker et al 2000; Barker 2003). Barker's hypothesis has inspired a number of research institutes around the world which now focus on the science of epigenetics, or how the environment to which we are exposed alters genes and therefore subsequent health and behaviour. The future may also see epigenetic research that demonstrates a greater understanding of the Oxytocin mediated calm and connection system and how normal birth is essential for its optimum functioning.

These examples are provided by way of support for the hypotheses explored here in relation to the plasticity of the developing fetus, infant and child. Clearly perinatal experiences can manipulate the genetic makeup of the developing human. This understanding is pivotal to midwifery care of childbearing women. Disrupting the normal Oxytocin pathways during the perinatal period may also impact the genetic blueprint of the fetus/infant.

One further confirmation of intergenerational changes in behaviour facilitated by Oxytocin is provided by research reported by two North American researchers (Pederson and Boccia 2002) who have described research conducted with female rats. Several interrelated findings from their studies indicate that the amount of maternal behaviour the rats receive from their own mothers in infancy is positively related to the development of Oxytocin receptor areas of the adult brain where Oxytocin stimulates maternal behaviour or diminishes anxiety and responses to stress. When these rats became mothers themselves, their maternal behaviour towards their pups positively correlated with their own received maternal behaviours and stress responses. This strongly suggests that Oxytocin has facilitated permanent brain changes. The implications of these findings for midwifery practice will be discussed below.

THEORY FOR CREATING AND MAINTAINING SAFE BIRTH SPACES

Natalie Angier, a medical journalist, describes birth as a '... feat of almost cataclysmic stress' (Angier 1999, p. 308). How do women manage to deal with this high level of stress? The answer lies with Oxytocin. The stress of birth could be called the midwife to devotion since stress activates Oxytocin which in turn facilitates a strong bond between the mother and her infant; enables the mother to conserve energy to produce sufficient calories for her baby's growth; calms the mother and slows her down so that she enjoys the enforced period of stillness required for breastfeeding and caring for her infant; increases the mother's sociability so that she seeks and attracts other companions to help with the care of her infant and herself, and ultimately improves the long-term physical and emotional health of both the mother and her infant.

Stress sets the neurophysiological stage for attachment says Angier. Women anticipating birth may be overcome by a sense of panic and foreboding and they seek the company of others to provide support and companionship. For women, the thought of giving birth alone is terrifying, unlike animals who seek solitude. Among humans birth is a shared experience. Importantly the chemistry of stress bears its own relief in a neurochemical antidote to female anxiety, the neuro-hormone Oxytocin, helping the mother conserve energy, and experience less pain, less anxiety, greater calmness and readiness to greet the new baby with open heart and mind (Angier 1999).

Throughout this chapter I have examined research that demonstrates women's response to stress may not be the automatic 'flight or flight' response seen in men, but is more likely to be the 'calm and connection' system integrated by Oxytocin. The research reviewed has provided ample evidence of the potential permanent consequences of disrupting the normal female stress response process during childbirth with impacts on both physiology and behaviour. The genetic blueprint is plastic. Environmental variations switch on and/or off parts of the genome resulting in a variety of outcomes. Oxytocin, endogenous opioid mechanisms and oestrogen are not the only neurohormones that play a role in behaviour. Future research will reveal more and we need to be able to access new knowledge and understandings as they emerge. But our ability to do that is limited by the dominant mechanistic medical model of childbirth that sees bodies as operating independently of minds – the so-called Cartesian dualism. We are stuck in naïve and mechanistic modes of practice and research. Therefore we need new approaches that utilize all the new understandings of the integrated and inseparable mind/body.

The implications of these findings are profound for midwives and all health-care providers who work with childbearing women since these findings have implications for society as a whole. We can no longer fail to adequately consider the dynamic nature of prenatal and perinatal life for moulding the future person and member of our community.

We need to consider very carefully how midwifery is involved in the shaping of the future. This raises a number of research and practice imperatives that will be examined in the final section of this chapter.

CREATING SAFE BIRTH SPACES

Understanding the Oxytocin system is a key to approaching the creation of safe birth spaces since it is the agent behind all states of relaxation and wellbeing. Integrating this knowledge into midwifery education, practice and research will enable a new approach to childbirth that optimizes the possibility for healthy, normal, safe and satisfying birth experiences. These kinds of birth experiences are not only essential for the long-term health of individuals but also for the health of society as a whole.

Translating this knowledge into midwifery practice
Oxytocin is stimulated in response to suckling during breastfeeding and during labour but we now know that Oxytocin is also stimulated by non-noxious stimulation; through touch, warmth, and stroking using light pressure (effluage). Touch can be external, stimulating the fibres of our greatest touch organ, the skin; or internal through stimulating the gastro intestinal system. Touch occurs during interaction with others; close individual contact, or pleasant social contact or through ritualized or formalized contact such as massage. Table 5.2 provides a summary of what is currently known about Oxytocin that is of particular relevance to birth and parenting, and midwifery practice. These effects are both physiological and behavioural. This knowledge is foundational for optimal midwifery practice and examples of its application in practice are provided in the following section.

Labouring undisturbed
The concept of labouring undisturbed is complex since it incorporates experiences and expectations of the woman that have possibly already

Table 5.2 Summary of Oxytocin (by itself or in interaction with other neuro-hormones) with particular relevance to birth and parenting

Oxytocin effects on physiology and behaviour	Initiates and maintains bonding, attachment and love
	Increases trust
	Improves social cohesion through decreasing aggression
	Conserves energy
	Induces sleep
	Stimulates growth and development and aids digestion
	Improves memory and aids learning
	Increases pain threshold
	Integrates endorphin/opiate system and a number of other neuro-chemical biological systems
	Improves healing
	Increases activity of immune system
	Lowers blood pressure
	Lowers heart rate
	Lowers level of stress hormones
	Stimulates contraction of myometrium (uterine muscle)
	Stimulates contractions of lactiferous ducts and alveoli of the breast
Oxytocin can be stimulated by:	Love (sense of being loved and loving towards others)
	Smell (aromatherapy)
	Touch – of particular pressure and rhythm and rate (40' beats per minute)
	Touch of naked skin on skin
	Touch in particular places (back, shoulders, arms in humans – front of body in animals)
	Touching others (hugs, hand on shoulder, massaging others, shaking hands)
	Touching the breasts and breastfeeding
	Eye-to-eye contact
	Massage
	Acupuncture, acupressure
	Eating
	Suckling (even non-nutritive suckling)
	Warmth
	Immersion in warm water
	Being in the company of known (and trusted) and pleasant companions
	Hearing pleasant sounds
	Seeing scenes of nature, in particular water
	Stretching of the vagina (as in the Ferguson reflex)
	Sexual activity
	Assuming particular facial and postural characteristics (smiles)
	Relaxing activities (meditation, hypnosis, playing, singing)
	Imagining pleasant/loving situations
	Nor-adrenaline
Oxytocin can be blocked by:	Artificial oxytocin (induced or augmented labour)
	Anaesthetics (epidural, pudendal block)
	Analgesics
	Caesarean birth
	Failure to stimulate the Ferguson reflex
	Adrenaline/fear
	Artificial feeding
	Atosiban (Oxytocin antagonist)
	Distracting the neocortex from its primary birth focus (e.g. engaging the mother in chatting about external, irrelevant events during labour)
	Feeling uncared for, disrespected
	Unsupportive companions
	Separation of mother and baby at birth
	Stressful experiences and expectations
	Hostile environments

(continued)

Table 5.2   Summary of Oxytocin (by itself or in interaction with other neuro-hormones) with particular relevance to birth and parenting—Cont'd

Blocking Oxytocin may result in:	Altered neuro-anatomy*
	Altered immune system (disorders)
	Operative birth (augmented labour, forceps, ventouse, caesarean section)
	Failed breastfeeding
	Upregulation of stress response
	Hypertension
	Hypervigilance (post-traumatic stress disorder)
	Type 1 diabetes
	Depression
	Autism
	Schizophrenia
	Cancers
	Cardiovascular disease
	Polycystic ovaries
	Genetic changes*
	Inability to love oneself or others
	Criminal and antisocial behaviour

*These changes may be permanent and may persist for generations if the neuro-anatomy or genetic structure of the individual is altered by switching on or off particular genes.

influenced her developing baby and the course of labour, before labour starts. We need therefore to establish models of care that enable women and midwives (or other carers) to meet before conception, provide care throughout pregnancy and during labour and the early postnatal experience of mother and baby, if we are to be able to ensure that the bio-behavioural Oxytocin system is able to function optimally.

While the effectiveness of 'continuity of midwifery care' has been well-established for more than a decade now, very few of us work in this model of care or anything that even approaches it. We need a renewed commitment to true continuity of care as the most common model of midwifery practice. Continuity of midwifery care provides opportunities for the calm and connection system to be unconsciously activated and optimized, leading to a safe birth without unnecessary intervention, to improve short-term and long-term health for both the mother and her baby. Importantly, continuity of midwifery care enables the baby's father and other family members who are part of his/her environment, to be integrated into the calm and connection system ensuring the ongoing health of the whole family and ultimately society.

In order that prenatal expectations are realistic and that women anticipating pregnancy have

an opportunity to understand the vitally important life transition they are about to experience, midwives need to extend their practice to the provision of information to young men and women in secondary schools and in pre-conception counselling. With women delaying pregnancy until their 30s there are many opportunities for this to occur.

Optimizing the environment for undisturbed labour means paying attention to the physical and metaphysical/spiritual spaces in which labour and birth occur at home, in hospitals and birth centres. Chapter 7 reveals more detail about an optimal birth environment where a woman feels in control, safe, secure, uninhibited and free to move with the rhythm of her body in a responsive way. The space provides key elements such as a lockable outer door to guarantee the woman's privacy; opportunities to see and experience warm water; comfortable furniture; quietness and birth companions such as midwives who know how to optimize the Oxytocin system.

Using the senses to enhance Oxytocin release

Optimizing midwives are knowledgeable and skilled professionals who have an established and trusting relationship with the woman; they are confident in her ability to birth; they speak in quiet and respectful ways in voices that are low pitched and therefore reassuring and calming. Considering all the ways in which the Oxytocin system can be enhanced through stimulation of our senses provides many opportunities for practice, for example stimulating touch senses through massage (at 40 beats per minute) and acupuncture or acupressure; warm water immersion or showering or simple hot, wet nappies applied to the woman's back; stimulating internal touch (the gut) through the provision of sweetened foods or fluids; stimulating the sexual release of Oxytocin through encouraging the couple to touch – skin to skin, hug and kiss (hence the lockable door to ensure privacy); through the provision of respect and genuine interest and care in the woman's wellbeing at all times.

Understanding the ways in which Oxytocin can be blocked and what the consequences might be for the long-term health of both mother and baby, will enable midwives to work to provide women with alternatives to inducing or augmenting labour with *artificial oxytocin*. This will also mean providing pain relief options for women that do not include opiates or anaesthetic agents and promoting them positively and respectfully. Changing practice to focus on new ways of caring for women will inevitably mean that we will be challenged to provide the evidence on which new practices are based. The result will be that midwives will be able to skillfully access the many research databases that exist (and are constantly being updated), in order to seek out and provide, interpret and apply the evidence. Some of that evidence has been examined in this and in other chapters of the book as a starting place.

Ensuring that the labouring woman's neocortex is not distracted from its primary focus of giving birth is also paramount. For midwives this means developing an awareness of the state of 'flow' that the woman exhibits. Flow is the name given to the bio-behavioural state that an athlete experiences when focused on the goal of achieving some physical feat. Labouring women are similarly goal oriented, with their whole mind/body intent on achieving a profoundly life changing physical and emotional process. Nothing should distract the woman from this primary purpose, so an optimizing midwife will think ahead before asking questions or engaging the woman in side conversations and will also encourage this behaviour in the woman's birth companions. People will not walk in and out of the birth room, but will be a constant supportive presence. If in a hospital, external noises such as machinery or metallic sounds suggestive of hard-edged technology; loudspeakers and paging systems; the sounds of other women in labour; will all be masked so as not to intrude on the woman's sense of purpose and calmness.

Once the baby is born, the optimizing midwife will ensure the baby is placed skin to skin on the mother's chest and when mother and baby have had time to meet and rest a while, will ensure the baby is given the opportunity to suckle at his/her mother's breast. This is best to happen before the mother has washed in order that the baby's smell receptors are stimulated, enhancing the baby's ability to find the nipple and latch effectively which is so important for successful breastfeeding to occur, but equally importantly, for attachment to be facilitated. (I often reflect on my time on the postnatal ward as a student midwife, carefully instructing women in how to wash and dry their nipples before attempting to breastfeed and did not pause to wonder why I soon provided bottles of artificial formula to their crying infants.)

These are just a few of the many ways that the knowledge and understanding of Oxytocin mediated bio-behavioural states can be translated into midwifery practice.

Translating this knowledge into midwifery education

A revolution happened in biology with the discovery of DNA in 1953 and the subsequent mapping of the human genome. It is a revolution with which our education system has not kept pace and it is clearly important that we catch up quickly. It was thought that the human genome project would identify around 140,000 genes since there are around that number of proteins that are required to sustain life as we know it (genes contain the DNA/protein blueprints). Imagine the shock of discovering that there are only around 34,000 genes to account for the amazing diversity of people and populations that exist around the world (Lipton 2005).

The conclusion reached by the scientific community was that it cannot be the DNA in our genes that is the sole source of controlling our biology and behaviour. The idea of genetic determinism was undone. It seems that there exists another process that involves switching on and off particular genes to account for human diversity in biology and behaviour. Scientists are now discovering what it is that controls the gene switches. Several important writers in the field of biology, physiology and psychology propose that the process that initiates that flick of the switch is our understanding of the environment that we need to adapt to at any given time and that *environment is perceived through our senses* (Pert 1997; Rossi 2002; Ridley 2004; Lipton 2005). Therefore sensory perception is the key to our physiology and behaviour.

The education syllabus for preparing midwives for practice needs to be reconstructed with an enhanced understanding of the maternal environment for the developing baby as the central focus. The periconceptual and perinatal environment for the woman is crucially important and the midwifery relationship with the woman is an important element of that environment. This information is not a 'nice to know' but is the underpinning rationale and understanding of the purpose of midwifery and how it should be enacted to promote normal birth. A transdisciplinary approach to knowledge for midwifery education and practice needs to be the basis of our education syllabus. This means having academics prepared in knowledge fields as diverse as anthropology, biology, epidemiology, nutrition, genetics, sociology and psychology (to name a few). We need to reconsider the current biomedical, pathological and primitive mechanical focus on birth and place it in the context of this more detailed understanding of optimal healthy childbirth. If we are to earn the title of 'expert in the normal' then we need to focus on normal childbearing in every aspect of educational preparation – with a neuro-hormonal and physiological focus.

We need to reconsider the belief that *exogenous oxytocin* used to induce or augment labour is innocuous. We need to reflect on the impact of disrupting Oxytocin pulsatile release which is a consequence of caesarean section birth. We need to use the knowledge that infant formulae do not contain bioactive hormones or growth factors, and artificial feeding is a potential hormonal manipulation that may have serious consequences ranging from impacts on brain growth to later stress reactivity in the infant and child and later, the adult (Carter 2003). Our midwifery education system requires the teaching of birth as much more than a mechanical process but see it as a complex integration of mind/body chemicals of emotion which aim to conserve the mother's energy so that she can welcome and nurture a new being.

Exploring this knowledge in midwifery research
While many of these new interpretations and understandings of the periconceptual and perinatal environment are still largely at the level of theoretical knowledge; extrapolating from animal research to human physiology and behaviour; we can now use these theoretical propositions as the justification for a range of research possibilities.

As Carter (2003) suggests, we need more animal studies that investigate the potential long-term behavioural consequences of *exogenous oxytocin* use during childbirth and long-term exposure to endogenous Oxytocin in prolonged and difficult labour. We need to encourage the development of more refined methods for the detection of Oxytocin so that we can find proof that the fetus is not influenced during administration of the hormone to mothers. We need more sophisticated research into the differences in human milk and formula and the long-term impact in terms of infants whose peptide history is manipulated through artificial feeding. We need research to determine whether the acute stress response in healthy mothers and babies during unmedicated birth may have positive or negative consequences on infant health (Bell and McFarlin 2006).

One group of researchers has already established that the number of Oxytocin receptors in the uterine muscle may be highly variable among women (Rezapour et al 1996). In a study of 50 women who were undergoing caesarean section for a variety of reasons, small pieces of uterine muscle were obtained and analysed. Women who had not laboured at all and those who received a caesarean section following 'failure to progress' had a smaller number of Oxytocin receptors. The implications are clear. Future research might include questions such as, would oxytocin-mediated behaviours included in pregnancy care increase the likelihood of normal birth (e.g. regular touch massage to increase either Oxytocin production or the development of larger numbers of Oxytocin receptors)? A pilot study for a randomized controlled trial of regular massage during pregnancy has been recently published so it is encouraging to see that this is not an isolated thought but that other midwives are actively pursuing these research ideas too (McNabb et al 2006).

Studies could be undertaken to determine if pregnancy loss was affected by the nature of the periconceptual emotional environment on the part of both parents; randomized controlled trials of therapies such as hypnosis or visualization could be undertaken to determine the impact of mental processes on a range of pregnancy outcomes such as induction of labour, labour progress and birth; continuous touch in labour could be explored to determine its impact on outcomes; acupuncture and acupressure are all deserving of systematic examination; the nature of the physical birth space of particular dimensions and incorporating particular principles and their impact on women's perceptions of safety could tell us a lot about how such spaces influence birth processes and outcomes. Useful studies would determine the characteristics of the optimizing midwife so that these characteristics could better inform educational preparation for midwifery practice. We need more studies to determine the most effective models of continuity of midwifery care that simultaneously ensure optimal outcomes for mothers and babies but that also support midwives in healthy work/life balance. Research needs to be undertaken with women who have experienced a caesarean birth to determine the impact of Oxytocin enhancing behaviours on breastfeeding (such as naked skin-to-skin contact for certain periods – one mother has revealed that getting into the bath and while wet, having the wet naked baby placed on her chest made her feel as if she had just given birth vaginally and an overwhelming sense of

love and attachment to her baby occurred); determining the impact of Oxytocin enhancing behaviours on women seeking vaginal birth after caesarean needs to be considered.

I am sure that many other research ideas have occurred to you as you have read this chapter and others. There are many possibilities.

CONCLUSION

It is now time to return to the questions posed at the beginning of this chapter.

- What is normal birth?
- Why do we need to promote normal birth?
- How will the future of education, practice and research be shaped by a new understanding of normal birth?

Normal birth is a complex process. It is much more than the simple mechanical act portrayed by textbooks which describe the powers, the passenger and the process. Oxytocin has a far larger role to play than merely stimulating the uterus to contract and breastmilk to pour into the baby's mouth. We need to write new textbooks that appreciate the true nature of Oxytocin and the ways in which it orchestrates every aspect of the mother's mind/body to conceive, to nourish the growing baby, to give birth, and to produce milk and love to nurture the new person. We need new textbooks that explore the long-term impacts of Oxytocin and Oxytocin-induced behaviours on our genetic blueprint.

Some of the evidence provided in this chapter has revealed ways in which normal birth can become disturbed by what is perceived as a hostile birth environment. The perception of 'hostility' can be something as subtle as an uncaring or unkind word on entering the birth space; feeling alone and not connected to others in the childbirth space; failing to touch in a particular way that the mother finds comforting. Women and babies may be exposed to unnecessary risks through the application of *exogenous oxytocin* to speed up labour; through an epidural or caesarean delivery; by separating the baby from its mother in the first moments of birth; by failing to facilitate the act of suckling and failing to consider that this is more than simply calorie-seeking behaviour.

We need to promote and protect normal birth simply because the future of humanity depends on it. Our ability to love is nurtured in the womb and can be altered at any time-up until the passing of puberty – by the perception of a hostile environment that switches on or off critical genes. This chapter has explored some of the consequences of exposure to events that lead to an impaired ability to love oneself or others.

As midwives we carry a huge responsibility to disseminate this knowledge to women so that they can make truly informed decisions about what procedures they will accept or seek during pregnancy and childbirth and breastfeeding. Midwives who understand the importance of not disturbing normal physiology and who work to protect undisturbed birth are the true guardians of the birth territory.

References

Adamsons K, Mueller-Heubach E, Myers R 1971 Production of fetal asphyxia in the rhesus monkey by administration of catecholamines to the mother. American Journal of Obstetrics and Gynecology 109(2): 248–262.

Angier N 1997 Bonobo society: Amicable, amorous and run by females. New York Times April 22.

Angier N 1999 Woman. An intimate geography. Houghton Mifflin, New York.

Arseneault L, Cannon M, Poulton R, Murray R, Caspi A, Moffitt T 2002 Cannabis use in adolescence and risk for adult psychosis: longitudinal prospective study. British Medical Journal 325: 1212–1213.

Barker D 1998 Mothers, babies and health in later life. Churchill Livingstone, London.

Barker D, Shiell A, Barker M, Law V 2000 Growth in utero and blood pressure levels in the next generation. Journal of Hypertension 18(7): 843–846.

Barker D 2003 The developmental origins of adult disease: Editorial. European Journal of Epidemiology 18: 733–736.

Bell A, McFarlin B 2006 Maternal and fetal stress responses during birth: Adaptive or maladaptive? Journal of Midwifery and Women's Health 51(5): 319–320.

Carter C 2003 Developmental consequences of oxytocin. Physiology and Behaviour 79: 383–397.

Carter C, DeVries A, Getz I 1995 Physiological substrates of mammalian monogamy: the prairie vole model. Neuroscience and Biobehavioral Reviews 19(2): 303–314.

Curtis J, Liu Y, Wang K 2001 Lesions of the vomeronasal organ disrupt mating-induced pair bonding in female prairie voles (Microtus ochragaster). Brain Research 18: 901(1–2): 164–174.

Cushing B, Carter C 2000 Peripheral pulses of oxytocin increase partner preferences in female, but not male, prairie voles. Hormones and Behavior 37(1): 49–56.

Da Costa A, Guevara-Guzman C, Rosalinda G, Ohkura Satoshi, Goode J, Kendrick K 1996 The Role of oxytocin release in the paraventricular nucleus in the control of maternal behaviour in the sheep. Journal of Neuroendocrinology 8(3): 163–177. Online. Available doi: 10.1046/j.1365–2826.1996.04411.x.

De Waal F 1995 Bonobo sex and society. The behavior of a close relative challenges assumptions about male supremacy in human evolution. Scientific American 82–88.

El-Hamamy E, Arulkumaran S 2005 Poor progress of labour. Current Obstetrics and Gynaecology 15(1): 1–8.

Foureur M 2005 Next Steps: public health in midwifery practice. In: P O'Luanaigh, C Carlson (Eds). Midwifery and Public Health: Future directions and new opportunities. Elsevier, Oxford.

Foureur M, Hunter M 2006 The place of birth. In: S Pairman, J Pincombe, C Thorogood, S Tracey (Eds). The midwifery textbook, 1st Australian and New Zealand edn. Elsevier, Australia.

Geary D, Flinn M 2002 Sex differences in behavioural and hormonal response to social threat: Commentary on Taylor et al 2000. Psychological Review 109: 745–750.

Gimpl G, Fahrenholz F 2001 The Oxytocin receptor system: Structure, function, and regulation. Physiological Reviews 81: 629–683.

Hutton J 1986 The problem patient. Induction and augmentation of labour. Current Therapeutics 61–74.

International Confederation of Midwives 2005 Definition of The Midwife. ICM Council Meeting 19th July Brisbane Australia. Online. Available http://www. internationalmidwives.org

Kendrick K, Keverne E, Baldwin B 1987 Intracerebroventricular oxytocin stimulates maternal behaviour in the sheep. Neuroendocrinology 46(1): 56–61.

Krehbiel D, Poindron P, Lev F, Prud'Homme M 1987 Peridural anaesthesia disturbs maternal behaviour in primiparous parturient ewes. Physiology and Behavior 40 (4): 463–472.

Lipton B 2005 The biology of belief. Mountain of Love/Elite Books, California.

Malhotra A, Kestler L, Mazzanti C, Bates J, Goldberg T, Goldman D 2002 Functional polymorphism in the COMT gene and performance on a test of prefrontal cognition. American Journal of Psychiatry 159: 652–654.

McNabb M, Kimber L, Haines A, McCourt C 2006 Does regular massage from late pregnancy to birth decrease maternal pain perception during labour and birth? A feasibility study to investigate a programme of massage, controlled breathing and visualization from 36 weeks of pregnancy until birth. Complementary Therapies in Clinical Practice 12(3): 222–231.

Mead M 1966 The diagnosis of foetal distress: A challenge to midwives. Journal of Advanced Nursing 23: 975–983.

Mongan M 2005 Hypnobirthing. Health Communications, Florida.

Naaktgeboren C 1989 The biology of childbirth. In: I Chalmers, M Enkin, M Keirse (Eds). Effective care in pregnancy and childbirth, Vol 1. Oxford University Press, Oxford.

Nathanielsz P 1992 Life before birth and a time to be born. Promethean Press, New York.

Newton N, Foshee D, Newton M 1966a Experimental inhibition of labor through environmental disturbance. Obstetrics and Gynecology 27(3): 371–376.

Newton N, Foshee D, Newton M 1966b Parturient mice: Effects of environment on labor. Science 151(3717): 1560–1561.

Newton N, Peeler D, Newton M 1968 Effect of disturbance on labor: Experiment using one hundred mice with dated pregnancies. American Journal of Obstetrics and Gynecology 8: 1096–1102.

Newton N 1972 The point of view of the consumer. From the Proceedings of the National Congress on the Quality of Life. In: N Newton 1990 On birth and women. Birth and Life Bookstore, Seattle.

Newton N 1986 Special Issues in nurse-midwifery: A look at the past and future. Journal of Nurse Midwifery 31(5): 232–239.

Newton N 1990 Newton on Birth and Women. Selected Works of Niles Newton, both classic and current. Birth and Life Bookstore. Seattle, Washington.

Nissen E, Gustavsson P, Widstrom A, Uvnäs-Moberg K 1998 Oxytocin, prolactin, milk production and their relation with personality traits in women after vaginal delivery and Sectio Casearean. Journal of Psychosomatic Obstetrics and Gynecology 19: 49–58.

Odent M 1999 The scientification of love. Free Association Books, London.

Pederson C, Boccia M 2002 Oxytocin links mothering received, mothering bestowed and adult stress responses. International Journal on the Biology of Stress 5(4): 259–267.

Pert C 1997 The molecules of emotion: The science behind mind–body medicine. Scribner, New York.

Rezapour M, Backstrom T, Ulmsten U 1996 Myometrial steroid concentration and oxytocin receptor density in parturient women at term. Steroids 61(6): 338–344.

Ridley M 2004 Nature via nurture. Genes, experience and what makes us human. Harper Perennial, London.

Rossi E 2002 The psychobiology of gene expression. WW Norton, New York.

Rowley M, Hensley M, Brinsmead M, Wlodarcyzk J 1995 Continuity of care by a midwife team versus routine care during pregnancy and birth: A randomised trial. Medical Journal of Australia 163: 289–93.

Rowley M 1998 Evaluation of team midwifery care in pregnancy and childbirth: A randomised controlled trial. Unpublished PhD Thesis, University of Newcastle, NSW.

Segal S 2002 Epidural analgesia and the progress and outcome of labor and delivery. International Anaesthesiology Clinics 40(4): 13–26.

Segal S 2001 Anesthesia and the progress of labour. Canadian Journal of Anesthesia 48: R8.

Shnider S, Levinson G 1987 Anesthesia for obstetrics. Williams and Wilkins, Baltimore.

Simkin P 1986 Stress, pain and catecholamines in labor: Part 1. A review. Birth 13(4): 227–33.

Simkin P, Ancheta R 2000 The labor progress handbook. Blackwell Publishing, Oxford.

Sosa R, Kennell J, Klaus M, Robertson S, Urrutia J 1980 The effect of a supportive companion on perinatal problems, length of labor, and mother–infant interaction. New England Journal of Medicine 303(11): 597–600.

Taylor S, Klein L, Lewis B, Gruenewald T, Gurung R, Updegraff J 2000 Biobehavioural responses to stress in females: Tend-and-befriend, not fight-or-flight. Psychological Review 107: 411–429.

Teixeira J, Fisk N, Glover V 1999 Association between maternal anxiety in pregnancy and increased uterine artery resistance index: cohort based study. British Medical Journal 318: 153–157.

Uvnäs-Moberg K 2004 Massage, relaxation and well-being: A possible role for oxytocin as an integrative principle? In: T Field (Ed). Touch and massage in early child development. Johnson and Johnson Pediatric Research Institute.

Uvnäs-Moberg K 2003 The Oxytocin factor. Tapping the hormone of calm, love, and healing. Da Capo Press, Cambridge MA.

Uvnäs-Moberg K 1997 Physiological and endocrine effects of social contact. Annals of the New York Academy of Sciences 807(1): 146–163.

Verbalis J, McCann M, McHale C, Stricker E 1986 Oxytocin secretion in response to cholescystokinin and food: Differentiation of nausea from anxiety. Science 232: 1417–1419.

Williams J, Insel T, Harbaugh C, Carter C 1994 Oxytocin administered centrally facilitates formation of a partner preference in female prairie voles (*Microtus ochrogaster*). Journal of Neuroendocrinology 6(3): 2450–2467.

Chapter 6

The spiritual and emotional territory of the unborn and newborn baby

Carolyn Hastie

Her hands trembling, Jane slips the slim plastic object from its envelope. She carefully reads the instructions on the enclosed leaflet. Her eyes are fixed on the little round window as she delicately and deliberating puts one drop of the clear fluid on the window. How long does she have to wait? Each moment seems an eternity. Finally, a thin blue line appears across the window. Confirmed. Jane is pregnant. With that moment, a cocktail of hormones and electrical impulses flood and sweep through Jane and the cells of her developing pregnancy. Whatever Jane's reaction, be it fear, joy, elation, love, despair or a mixture of all these, a chain of physiological events will be released throughout her entire being. She will not be the only one who feels these feelings because her body is not one but two. For the rest of the pregnancy everything Jane thinks, feels, experiences and expresses will affect every part of both Jane and her unborn baby.

INTRODUCTION

Nature is always seeking to express itself. Everywhere we look there is evidence of the profusion of life. Farmers know when conditions are favourable, the harvest is bountiful. The natural world has an innate, constantly evolving blueprint for creating, growing, developing and reproducing itself. Scientific understanding about the complexity of life is also growing and developing. Scientific perceptions are shifting from the limitations imposed by the fixed, mechanical Newtonian view of a material universe which contains solid structures and empty space to that of quantum physics, which explains the cosmos as an intelligent, conscious, self-aware, interconnected, vibrating field of possibilities and information. In the quantum physics view, matter and energy are interchangeable. The cosmos and everything in it is constantly creating, adjusting and changing in response to environmental signals. From this perspective, health and disease relate to how the cells in the body interact with each other and their environment. This means that all phenomena, including pregnancy and birth involves a process of co-creation as consciousness, energy and information interact and coalesce into matter and experience (Lipton 2005).

Across disciplines, it is becoming more and more accepted that the womb is the crucible within which the foundation of health, intelligence, happiness, personality, sexuality and behaviour of the emerging person is forged (Speyrer 1995; Chamberlain 1998). Understanding what constitutes a favourable environment for optimal generation and procreation of human life is expanding. Knowledge about the effects of unfavourable environments is also expanding. Adequate nutrition and freedom from obvious teratogens, such as certain diseases, drugs and industrial chemicals are well known necessities. Less well known are the effects of the mother's emotional and spiritual life on the development of her baby. This chapter provides a beginning exploration of these effects. 'Mother as emotional and spiritual territory' of the unborn baby is explored from an integrated mindbodyspirit perspective. Until recently, spirit and emotions have been largely excluded from scientific and medical considerations. Ideas emerging from the science of quantum physics are bringing mind and body back together and integrating an understanding of 'spirit' into new scientific discoveries. For the purpose of this chapter, 'spirit' means the animating life force in every body and is a neutral, expanding power (see Chapters 3 and 4 for further discussion). Conscious thinking is a spiritual activity and spiritual competence involves intentional use of constructive thinking skills to focus on desired outcomes. As well as incorporating insights from quantum physics, this chapter contains a brief overview of current research into genes, brains, emotions, cells, body regulatory processes and the effect of maternal stress on fetal development.

This chapter shows how a mother thinks, feels, is treated, nurtured and cared for during her whole childbearing experience is of vital importance.

 Practical strategies for midwives are suggested within the text and are provided in boxes with a symbol of Pinard's stethoscope (used by midwives for listening to baby's heartbeat) like this: I present my own experience to begin the discussion of how a woman's experience of pregnancy and birth has life long consequences not only for her own sense of self, but also the expression of her child's spirit in mind and body. My own pregnancies provided the springboard for my interest in understanding the way our spirit and emotions impact the way that unborn babies grow and develop. I wondered why some die without obvious reasons and others survive.

My story

'I began my midwifery training in 1973. Four months into the course, I discovered I was pregnant. In those days there was no maternity leave and in fact, we weren't allowed to work if we were pregnant. At any other time, I would have been happy about the baby, but I was distraught that I would have to leave midwifery. Just after I discovered I was pregnant, we were given our eviction notice from the house we were renting and my sister-in-law was killed in a motorbike accident. My husband and I were devastated, as were my parents-in-law. I felt sad for myself as I had lost a good friend and deeply sad for them. I kept asking myself 'what must it be like to lose a child?' My obstetrician never once asked me how I was, what was going on in my life, how I was coping or how I felt. Our visits were perfunctory, brief and focused on the physical check. One afternoon, I was so desperate to talk to someone, I drove 20 minutes to visit a doctor I thought would listen to me. I had met him during my midwifery training. It was the end of the day and he obviously wanted to get home. After a very quick conversation, he offered me Valium. Enraged, I left his surgery, without the Valium. At 36 weeks gestation, my baby was diagnosed as an intrauterine death. We had been unable to find a house to live in and were living in a tent in a caravan park. I was 'left' for two weeks to see if I would labour. I didn't. What I did do was become incredibly angry and resentful. Again, there was no one I could talk to.

Throughout the next year, I tried to get pregnant again. I gave up at the end of the year and took a new

My story   Continued

job as a nurse in a haematology ward. As soon as I started my new job, I became pregnant. I was very, deeply upset. I was angry that I had taken a whole year off work trying to get pregnant and then, just as I started a new job, along came a pregnancy! I felt indignant and tricked. The emotional roller coaster started again and carried me with it. Again, there was no one to help process the deep emotional turmoil and despair I was feeling. I gradually got used to the idea of being pregnant, but at 16 weeks gestation, I haemorrhaged and miscarried. It is tempting to want to attribute these events to mere bad luck. I did for years. However, we are now beginning to understand the impact of emotional distress on our bodies and on our developing babies.'

THE BIOLOGY OF EMOTION

At a biological level, emotions are messenger molecules which have a central and pivotal role in all aspects of human life and wellbeing (Rossi 2002). New brain imaging tools such as functional magnetic resonance imaging (fMRIs) and positron emission tomography (PET) are being used to map areas of the brain in different subjective emotional states (Rossi 2002). It has been discovered that emotional states are physiological and dynamically involved in every aspect of human biology and behaviour. Emotions are the regulators and central organising process of the whole nervous system and subconscious processes.

When people perceive and think, their nervous system fires and tiny messenger molecules called ligands are released (Goleman 1996; Pert 1997). Ligands are made of strings of amino acids and drift around in the extracellular fluid throughout the body. These tiny strings of amino acids are emotions and function as neurotransmitters, hormones or peptides depending on their location. These substances are the language of the subconscious. Every cell in every body, including mothers and their unborn babies, has millions of sensing scanners which are molecules of twisting, bending protein chains also made up of amino acids. These tiny little scanners are called receptors and hover in the oily cell membranes ready for their chemical

messages. Ligands dock in and out of their matching receptors on cells, like a key going into a lock. Drugs, toxins, including excess stress hormones and teratogens can also act as ligands (Pert 1997). When ligands dock, they transmit a chemical message to the cell and then move off to some other receptor on some other cell. These chemical messages translate into mood, behaviour and activity (Pert 1997).

Bodily sensations result from the interaction of neural network vibrations and the messenger molecules of emotions and are experienced as feelings. Emotions and feelings intertwine to give life richness, depth and meaning. Feelings provide guidance and stimulate action. 'Gut instinct' for example, is a message from the subconscious intelligence of the enteric nervous system. This feeling often provides a source of innate wisdom for the individual. Throughout pregnancy, the mother's emotional life is setting the foundations for her baby's emotional life, her baby's physiological regulatory processes and her baby's subconscious patterns of behaviour, including 'gut instinct'. If the mother is happy and feels supported, the baby is happy and in this emotionally stable state, the baby's physiological processes are forming in optimal adaptable and flexible ways providing a good start to life. Discomfort in the gut, such as 'colic' experienced by a newborn baby, may in fact be a signal that there is some disturbance in mother baby interaction. It is important to recognize that this is an indication that the mother needs more support and to ensure the mother is well nourished and rested and has adequate social and practical support through this particular phase of mother baby relationship development.

The entire body is a cooperative, fluid intelligence system modulated by messenger molecules (ligands) of emotion (Pert 1997; Chamberlain 1998; Lipton 2005). These ligands are involved in everything from genetic expression, cell function, division and repair to organ oxygenation and cognition. Living cells are information processors and problem solving systems which are constantly interacting with their environment (Rossi 2002; Lipton 2005). When a person has a negative reaction to something and becomes emotionally distressed, messenger molecules are released which disrupt genetic expression, cellular interactions and body functioning. For a developing baby, who can't escape from its environment, exposure to ligands generated by chronic or uncontrollable distress during pregnancy has profound effects on its cells and genetic expression. The actual effect depends on the gestation and the particular part of the baby being created when maternal distress occurs. For example, if kidneys are being developed, nephron generation stops as the unborn baby's creative intelligence is diverted to dealing with the threat posed to existing cells by a sudden increase of stress hormones.

Emotions have been undervalued in health services and especially maternity services. In fact, pregnant women who seek to have their emotional needs meet are often labelled 'selfish'. There is now compelling evidence that meeting childbearing women's emotional needs is a critical part of any maternity service. John Heron (1989) has outlined three core emotional needs which are common to every human being. These are the need for:

1. **Love:** to be loved and to love; to give and receive caring, affection, warmth, appreciation, support.
2. **Understanding:** to understand and be understood; to have a grasp of what is happening.
3. **Choice:** to choose and be chosen – to be able to take part in the decisions that affect our lives – to be chosen as someone special because of our own particular gifts or qualities.

Heron explained that when these needs are not met, people develop psychological defence mechanisms which disrupt relationships. New understandings from quantum physics, epigenetics, psychobiology, endocrinology and molecular biology show that not only do unmet emotional needs disrupt people-to-people relationships, they also influence our physiology and our genetic expression. Far from being some 'airy fairy' philosophical idea, feeling valued and cared for and having control over one's life has important biological consequences. Pregnant women who feel they have control over what happens to them have reduced levels of cortisols (the hormones we release when we are distressed) in their peripheral circulation. As a pregnant woman's sense of control is eroded, her levels of glucocorticoids

go up (Schulkin, Schmidt and Erikson 2005). Glucocorticoids in excess are toxic to developing brains and nervous systems.

One of the maxims I heard during my midwifery training was that 'worry is the work of pregnancy'. This statement is partly true but misses the point. The real work of pregnancy is coming to terms with, resolving and reframing the things that are worrying the woman. Pregnant women certainly do worry about whether their baby is going to be normal; that appears to be part of the developmental process of transforming into a mother. There are, in addition, an increasing number of social pressures on childbearing women which add to the 'worrying' load. Many of these social pressures are an unavoidable part of modern life. The process of talking through worries with someone the woman knows and trusts is crucial. Midwives are ideally situated to support women through this spiritually and emotionally transformative process.

Health services should:
- Provide holistic preconceptual and perinatal clinics in primary health care settings.
- Provide relationship based midwifery services where childbearing women can access one to one midwifery care.
- Provide ample opportunity for women and their partners to explore their feelings about pregnancy, birth and parenting with their midwives.

THE PHYSIOLOGY OF LOVE AND FEAR

Concern, worry, trust and happiness are physiologically different bio-behavioural states of the mind/body, modulated by molecules of emotion. These different bio-behavioural states can be classified into two broad domains. These domains encompass the spectrum of love and fear. Each domain has an emotional 'charge' gradient from high to low. For example, in the domain of fear, that gradient runs from a whole body state of abject terror which stimulates a total and compelling fight, freeze or flight response, to a state of arousal or curiosity which can manifest as 'butterflies' in the abdomen. In the domain of love, it ranges from that 'over the moon' rapturous euphoric feeling to the happy, relaxed 'flow' state.

The autonomic nervous system actively mediates the two bio-behavioural domains along a continuum between high alert and deep bliss. Fluctuations of arousal and relaxation are normal and an integral part of living. Our perceptual and thinking processes, both conscious and habitual, trigger our autonomic nervous system. Emotional responses dictate which bio-behavioural pathway dominates at any given moment. There are two branches of the autonomic nervous system, the parasympathetic (relaxation pathway) and the sympathetic (alert pathway). The love state is associated with the parasympathetic pathway. Coherence, calmness and wellbeing is the result. This is our social, relational state of being and is the most favourable state for healthy, happy human life and relationships. It is the bio-behavioural state necessary for optimal learning, growth, health and development. When a person is in this state, the physiology is bathed in oxytocins and endorphins: the hormones of love and good feelings. For a pregnant woman, the parasympathetic state of wellbeing means her developing baby is similarly awash with happy hormones (Uvnas-Moberg 2003; Uvnas-Moberg, Arn and Magnusson 2005) and development proceeds in optimal ways.

Fear, with its fight/flight/freeze response, is a survival mechanism. It fires up when a threat to the person's wellbeing is perceived. When danger is about, the sympathetic aspect of the autonomic nervous system is switched on. The sympathetic pathway is regulated through the spinal cord and shuts off the parasympathetic pathway. Messenger molecules of stress, such as corticotrophin-releasing hormone (CRH), adrenalins and glucocorticoids (cortisols) are associated with this mechanism and are useful for short term strength, immediate alertness and fighting power. In the long term, these substances disrupt learning, growth and development. In states of constant arousal and threat, neurotransmitter interactions are derailed, cognitive brain functions shut down, growth and development stop, digestion is abandoned, blood flow rerouted, immune system function disrupted, inflammatory responses are stimulated and cells are damaged (Wadhwa 2005). For pregnant women, not only are their bio-behavioural processes affected, their babies are trying to grow and develop in a very hostile environment.

Working with many different women in a relationship-based private midwifery practice, I discovered that how we think, feel, live and experience life has an enormous impact on health, babies' growth and development, births and lives generally. Recognition of the multiple influences on the birth process is encapsulated by my understanding that 'women birth how they live'. Women living calm, peaceful, loving lives have calm, peaceful loving births and relaxed babies. Even when women's lives are less than ideal, I have learnt that when women talk about their issues, feel heard, loved and supported, unhelpful emotional energy dissipates. It is also apparent that pregnant women who express their fears, doubts, worries and emotional pain and helped to focus on what they want are likely to have normal births and few medical interventions. They also have a low incidence of both hypertension in pregnancy and premature labour. They have calm, relaxed babies. On the other hand, those who deny and suppress their emotional needs and distress usually end up with complications and interventions. I was fascinated to read the work of Gayle Peterson and Lewis Mehl (Peterson 1981) as their research on how women's attitudes, beliefs and emotions influenced their childbearing experiences confirmed my observations.

Contemporary midwifery practice competencies now include:

- Advanced interpersonal skills.
- Reflective practice.
- Clinical supervision.

And require midwives to:

- Ask childbearing women how they feel and what's happening in their lives at every visit.
- Listen to women and ask strategic questions.
- Embody suggestions in Chapter 3 – Midwifery Guardianship.

PREGNANCY LOSS AS A PROTECTIVE MECHANISM

Recently, on a sunny Saturday morning as I was having morning tea with a colleague, I was talking through my thinking about the way emotions affect unborn babies and the birth process. A look of recognition flitted across her face. My words had triggered an important insight for her. Cynthia (not her real name) told me her story and gave me permission to share it.

Unexplained miscarriage has been linked to a Th1/Th2 cytokine imbalance at the feto-maternal interface suggesting immune rejection of the fetus by the mother (Sugiura-Ogasawara et al 2002). Immunological functions are influenced by various psychological factors and it is thought that the psycho-neuro-immuno-endocrine network contributes to miscarriage. This cascade of events would fit with both Cynthia's and my reactions to our unplanned pregnancies. Perhaps this mechanism explains the high rate of miscarriage for New York women after the attacks on the World Trade Centre on 9/11 (Lichtarowicz 2003). Dust and other environmental contaminants may have been contributing factors, but sympathetic pathway activation would have been high. There are also parallels to be drawn with pregnant women's experience in Gaza following Israel's sonic boom attacks in 2006. Doctors reported a rise in miscarriage, stillbirth and premature birth rates following the attacks (O'Loughin 2006).

Maternal malnutrition and psychological (emotional) stress take its toll and early pregnancy loss and premature birth are associated with these adverse conditions. Some researchers suggest that evolution of our species may have been served by pregnancy loss when nutritional resources were inadequate for maternal wellbeing (Power and Tardiff 2005). Perhaps this evolutionary mechanism is switched on along with the sympathetic nervous system when mothers have clear, unambiguous negative reactions to pregnancy, like Cynthia and I did or when environmental conditions, like New York after 9/11 and Gaza during the sonic boom attacks, are perceived as terrifyingly dangerous. Using an evolutionary perspective, pregnancy loss in adverse conditions can be seen as a way of protecting mothers from dangers associated with nutritional deficit; emotional costs of unwanted pregnancies and the extra physical risks and limitations pregnancy could pose in dangerous environments. Babies who survive violent, anxious or negative environments are more likely to be born with smaller forebrains and larger hindbrains (Chilton Pearce 2004). Forebrains are associated with conscious intelligence and hindbrains are associated with reflex survival behaviours. Perhaps these adaptive brain configurations equip babies with responses more likely to help them survive in their social world. Some postulate a link between a hostile prenatal environment and later suicidal and criminal behaviour (Grof 1985).

THE MATERIALIZING BABY

It used to be thought that prenatal babies floated in a dreamy idyllic world, free of worries, protected from any harm, growing and developing in a linear, genetically predetermined way. We now know this is not the case. Babies do not emerge at birth as blank slates ready to learn. From conception, babies are conscious beings who are constantly learning, developing and growing according to environmental conditions. Scientists mapping the human genome were surprised to find only about 34,000 genes, which are not enough to explain human complexity. Far from being fixed as previously thought, genes are not destiny. Genetic determinism has given way to an understanding that the human genome is fluid and accommodating to the environment. In the same way prices flicker on the stock exchange in response to market pressures, genes

---

Cynthia's story

Cynthia was distraught when she discovered she was pregnant. There was just no way she could bring herself to face having another baby. Angry and desperate, she told the baby she didn't want it and begged it to go. Cynthia was angry with her husband and told him so. She was depressed and angry for two weeks. Her mood gradually changed. Slowly she came to some resolution over the next month. One week later she began to haemorrhage and was devastated again. A miscarriage was diagnosed as inevitable. Cynthia was taken to the operating theatre for a D&C (dilatation and curettage of the uterus). She couldn't understand why she would miscarry just as she was starting to get used to the idea of being pregnant. After the surgery she was told that the baby had died a month ago.

get expressed, changed and subsequently inherited through their response to environmental signals. Recognition that environmental influences such as nutrition, stress and emotions lead to selection and modification of genes has led to a new field of biology called Epigenetics. The process of selecting the most appropriate genes for expression is called genomic imprinting. It occurs in the final stages of sperm and ovum maturation and throughout the baby's development (Lipton 2005). Regulatory proteins within each and every cell are constantly monitoring environmental conditions and choosing which non-dominant gene gets expressed while creating and fine tuning as many as 2000 or so variations from any single gene's blueprint (de Kloet et al 2005; Lipton 2005). This means that both parents are genetic engineers months before conception. Which genes are expressed in the developing sperm and ova is under the influence of the parents' bio-energetic fields prior to and at the moment of conception. Maternal and paternal bio-energetic fields include consciousness, emotions, biology, nutrition, beliefs, attitudes, behaviour, habits and broader social and cultural influences (Lipton 2005).

 Midwives can help parents-to-be create an optimal environment for germ cell production by explaining that what they drink and eat, whether they take drugs or not, how they exercise, how they relate to each other and how they think and feel about their moment to moment life experiences, influences the way genes express in the ovum and sperm. If they make health, happiness and overall wellbeing a priority, the ovum and sperm will contain genetic material that reflects that state of consciousness. If the parents-to-be smoke, drink, take drugs and have unhappy, troubled relationships, then genes will be expressed which have the best chance of helping the individual survive in those harsh conditions.

From conception onwards, the developing baby takes an active role in its own construction (Wadhwa 2005). This process is called autopoiesis (Rose 2006). How the baby materializes is through self-evolving systems which uses environmental signals to modulate genetic expression. Relying on its mother's perception of her experience, that is her thinking, emotional life, nutrition, activities, culture and behaviours, the materializing baby constantly adjusts by changing its physiology and genetics to assimilate these environmental signals. Evolution of this ability to integrate and adapt to prevailing environmental conditions provides the best chance of survival. It also provides a means of ensuring the individual fits into the family and environment it is being born into (Lipton 2005; Wadhwa 2005).

When a baby is conceived, the woman's subconscious intelligence swings into action. Through chemical and energetic 'language', news travels through her subconscious mind/body like wildfire. From molecule to molecule, cells and organs, her nervous system and regulatory processes are in communication. If a woman's subconscious processes welcome a baby, cellular and vascular changes at the site of implantation enable the developing blastocyst to establish itself. The outer cells of the blastocyst proliferate, sending tiny finger like projections into the soft, rich lining of the woman's uterus. The uterus responds by switching off what would otherwise be a rejection response since the baby's cells are different from the mother's own cells, because they also contain paternal genetic material. If the woman's subconscious processes are not welcoming to a baby then the woman's immune system can react to the blastocyst as if it were a virus-like invader, sending white blood cells to engulf it. Some blastocysts don't make this first hurdle. Those that do survive this primordial life and death struggle will have the experience imprinted in their cells as their first experiential 'memory'. Amazing as it sounds, psychobiology informs us that all cells, not only immune cells, have memories. The events that surround conception and implantation may provide 'forerunners for sensation, emotions and personality' that have lifelong effects (Verny and Weintraub 2002). With implantation, cells differentiate into germ cells; the building blocks for specific systems, tissues and organs. The inner layer, the endoderm will become the digestive system, the lungs and glands. The middle layer, the mesoderm gives rise to muscles, lymphatic system, blood and excretory system. The outer layer, the ectoderm becomes skin and the body wide nervous system (England 1996).

The common genesis for skin and nervous system gives some inkling as to why skin-to-skin experience for mothers and babies at birth is so vitally important. For babies, undisturbed skin to skin experience with its mother will trigger necessary kinaesthetic, visual, motor, auditory sensory, hormonal and electrical impulses, firing and wiring the baby's somatosensory neural networks. These networks form the basis of loving relationships with the affective aspects of trust, affection and intimacy. For the mother, skin to skin contact with her baby at birth triggers the highest levels of the love and attachment hormone, oxytocin, promoting attachment with the baby and triggering uterine activity which releases the placenta and controls bleeding.

At the end of the first month, the rudimentary scaffolding of the heart, cerebral brain, neural network, gut, spinal cord, muscles and sense organs are in place. By this time, the vascular system is spinning its thread throughout the tissues and the heart tube is beating rhythmically. Beginnings of central and peripheral nervous systems, immune and endocrine systems appear in the first few weeks of pregnancy. Forty-four days after conception, 99% of an unborn baby's muscles, complete with nerve and vascular supply, are present (Tsiaras 2002). The second month of life is the crucial month for organ development and body building. As different parts of the nervous system and body develop, genes are switched on for each new stage of development. Genes expect certain conditions for expression and depend upon these conditions for development. As each group of cells divide, the daughter cells are not exact copies. They vary slightly according to which of their genes are switched on or off in response to environmental cues. It is important for parents to understand the human body is not merely made up of discrete and individual functioning organs. The body is actually an integrated and fluid intelligence system which begins to function in harmony with all parts of itself from very early pregnancy (Pert 1997; Chamberlain 1998).

Midwives can help parents understand that the maternal environment provides the spiritual, emotional, sensory, nutritional and chemical material from which, using genetic information,

the unborn baby constructs its body and mind. How these processes unfold form the origins of the future child's personality and health.

During the first 15 weeks of gestation discrete patterns of movement erupt as body parts emerge. These behavioural patterns are indicative of whether or not the nervous system is growing and developing in the right way. Patterns include breathing, hiccoughs, arm, leg, mouth and tasting movements (Van den Bergh et al 2005). Budding arms and legs begin moving at about seven weeks gestation. Scientists wondered why movement occurred so early. It is now recognized that movement actually propels development of the different body parts. Growth follows function. Episodes of movement and activity are interspersed with resting phases. These cycles of resting and activity become increasingly associated with identifiable heart rate patterns and rapid eye movements (REM) (Porges et al 1999). As the unborn baby becomes more mature and closer to term, the rest–activity cycles, involving increasingly regulated sets of delicate, intricate neural networks and neurotransmitter interactions, develop into behavioural state sleep–wake cycles. These states are: quiet sleep, active sleep, quiet wakefulness and active wakefulness. They form the foundation for adult sleep–wake behaviour (Van den Bergh, Mulder Mennes and Glover 2005). Anyone who has looked into the eyes of an alert, attentive newborn will recognize the state of quiet wakefulness. This state is a state of pure conscious awareness. Environmental factors like maternal stress or maternal smoking disrupt the sleep–wake cycles before, during and after birth.

Midwives can draw attention to these states of the unborn and newborn baby and explain the growth and maturation of the nervous system. Beginning processes are not easy to perceive in unborn babies, but parents can be helped to understand them by midwives who draw attention to changing phenomena, such as movements, sleep patterns and hiccoughs. Parents can be helped to understand that they are teaching the unborn baby all about their lifestyle. Their baby's sleep wake patterns are being formed by the activity and rest cycle of the parents. Parents can be encouraged to spend a few minutes at the beginning and end of the day, when they are relaxed in bed, stroking the baby through the woman's abdomen, talking to and feeling loving towards their baby. As they do, they will discover that their baby becomes responsive to these times, moving in synchrony with their stroking movements.

While the central nervous system and the development of the cerebral brain has been the focus of a great deal of interest and research, the peripheral nervous system has its brains too. Here 'brain' is understood to mean a localized neural network that coordinates organs, tissues and cells at the local level and operate both independently of and cooperatively with the central nervous system via the vagal nerve. The scientific field of neurocardiology has emerged with recognition that the heart has a brain (Heartmaths 2002) and neurogastroenterology is the new discipline concerned with the brain in the gut (Gershon 1999). It makes sense from an evolutionary standpoint that vital functions such as circulation and digestion would keep their ability to self regulate even after organisms became more complex and developed a cerebral brain. For example, the gut has about 100 million neurons, including sensory and motor neurons, information processing circuits and glial cells, major neurotransmitters; dopamine, serotonin, acetycholine, nitric oxide and norephinephrine. Even benzodiazepines are found in the enteric nervous system. Given that 95% of the body's serotonin is made in the bowel (Gershon 1999), it is easy to see how chronic maternal prenatal stress could prime the unborn baby's enteric nervous system for a lifetime of malfunction.

The rapidly budding nervous system receptors for the unborn baby's emerging senses are registering and incorporating experiences and information. The somatic (bodily) aspect of the autonomic nervous system collects sensory experiences, which enter the central nervous system through the evolving reticular activating system (RAS) and are processed through the emotional processing part of the nervous system. The RAS is an interlacement of thousands of nerve fibres located in the cerebral trunk, linking the brain stem and emotional processing

areas with the right socio-emotional prefrontal cortex of the brain. The RAS is fully activated during the sensitive period immediately after birth (Lipton 2005). It is the receiving station for billions of bits of incoming and outgoing sensory and motor information streaming from internal and external sources. A large part of its role is regulating various levels of consciousness and maintaining vital functions (Carlson 2004). The increasingly complex nervous system expects sensory environmental signals and depends on these signals to trigger genetic instructions for the next phase of development (Schore 2002). As in gamete formation, the quality of the environmental signal will determine which gene will provide the blueprint for expression (Siegal 1999; Herlenius and Lagercrantz 2004).

THE EFFECT OF MATERNAL SPIRITUAL AND EMOTIONAL DISTRESS IN PREGNANCY ON DEVELOPING BABIES

Fetal programming is the process by which environmental conditions impact the unborn baby during sensitive periods of development causing permanent effects on structure, physiology and metabolism (Barker 1998). Barker (1998) was the first to suggest that adverse intrauterine conditions impacted upon unborn babies physical growth and development setting the stage for adult disease states. His ideas became known as the Barker Hypothesis. The concept of fetal programming can be extended to incorporate emotional and spiritual development of unborn babies too. Maternal perceptions, thinking and emotions set the foundations for the developing baby's physiological regulation, world view and intelligence.

An example of unborn babies reacting to maternal responses to environmental stimuli is the 'fetal fright' bradycardia (slow heart rate) noted as a response to an air raid during the gulf war reported by Yoles and colleagues (1993). Not only do unborn babies become bradycardic when there is short-term acute maternal anxiety, they also become quiet and stop moving. Their heart rates lose variability, which can be a sign of fetal distress. Glucocorticoids (cortisols) are secreted when a person perceives a loss of control in times of fear and anxiety. Glucocorticoids are multi modal messenger molecules which behave differently depending on context and body region. They influence cognitive, behavioural and physiological domains. When a person's perception of being out of control rises, fear and anxiety increases, leading to a corresponding swell in the levels of glucocorticoids. When there is a perception of control, there is a corresponding reduction in free circulating glucocorticoids (Schulkin et al 2005).

 Midwives can help pregnant women maintain control. Strategies include:

- Supporting women to get their emotional needs met.
- Providing evidence based information.
- Ensuring women have choice about what happens to them throughout their childbearing experience and how midwives can support their decisions.
- Explaining physiology of emotions and role of autonomic nervous system.
- Discuss ways to deal with fear, anxiety and tension, thereby reducing sympathetic pathway activation. Strategies include:
  - deep breathing
  - conscious relaxation strategies
  - sitting quietly, focusing on the baby
  - talking to the baby about what is happening in the mother's life
  - self nurturing activities: massages, good food, exercise, rest etc
  - referral to counselling services as appropriate.

The adverse effects of poor nutrition, drugs, alcohol, smoking and environmental chemicals on developing babies are well known. Messenger molecules associated with maternal emotional distress are increasingly gaining attention as another form of environmental toxicity. Evidence is mounting that when a pregnant woman lives with chronic levels of distress, or has a severe acute stressful experience, fetal development is compromised. Excess stress hormones have been shown to disrupt the genomic imprinting process and even switch it off altogether causing disease, aberrant growth and abnormal morphology of the unborn baby (Hansen et al 2000; Wadhwa 2005; Power and Schulkin 2005).

Both the mother herself and her unborn baby are adversely affected by the actions of elevated levels of stress related hormones, peptides and immune system cells in pregnancy. The following list highlights some of the effects associated with these substances:

For the mother:

- Abnormal labour, dystocia and higher rates of maternal morbidity (Saunders et al 2006).
- Birth interventions and analgesia (Jacobsen et al 987; Raine et al 1997).
- Reduced colostral beta endorphin galactopoiesis (Zanardo et al 2001).

For her unborn baby:

- Miscarriages, stillbirths, premature births and congenital abnormalities (Hansen et al 2000; Nepomnaschy et al 2006; O'Loughlin 2006).
- Alterations to normal functioning in all nervous system regulatory and neurotransmitter systems of babies, including opioid, cholinergic, serotonergic, dopaminergic, GABA-ergic and noradrenergic systems (Mulder et al 2002).
  - Disturbances in maturing sleep wake cycle networks – characteristic of neurological and psychopathological disease, such as autism, depression and schizophrenia (Huizink et al 2004).
  - Compromised normal regulation of placentally derived corticotrophin-releasing-hormone (CRH) and/or cortisol associated with impaired habituation to environmental stimuli of unborn baby and temperamental difficulties in infants. Predisposition to attention deficits and depressive illness (Welberg and Secki 2001; Weinstock 2005).
  - Increased uterine artery resistance index – associated with low birth weight and adult disease states (Teixeira et al 1999).
  - Broad range of physical, emotional, cognitive and behavioural problems in childhood such as: reduced attention span, ADHD, aggression, impulsivity and anxiety (Van den Bergh et al 2005).
  - Learning difficulties (Lemaire et al 2000).
- Health and behaviour adversely affected by hypothalamic-pituitary-adrenal axis (HPA),

peripheral nervous system, autonomic nervous system dysregulation (O'Connor et al 2005; Van den Bergh et al 2005; Saunders et al 2006).

– Individuals with hyperactivated and dystregulated HPA axis react more rapidly and dramatically to stressful events and stay upset for longer than those with a normally regulated HPA (Mulder et al 2002; Matthews 2002; Austin et al 2005).

– Psychopathology in later life (Lemaire et al 2000).

- High impulsivity during performance on cognitive tasks in 14 and 15-year-olds (Van den Bergh et al 2005).
- Elevated cortisol production in adolescence and tendency to behavioural difficulties and depression (O'Connor et al 2005).
- Alterations in social and sexual behaviour (Mastorakos et al 2006).
- Delayed motor development; reduced ability to adapt to new and different situations; blunted curiosity – characteristics which persist in adulthood (Mulder et al 2002).
- Acute maternal stress between 21–32 weeks gestation is associated with autism (Beversdorf et al 2005).
- Increased movements and reduced heart rate variability (Panksepp 2001).

– Increased risk of heart disease and diabetes in later life associated with prolonged fetal heart rate reactions (Van den Bergh et al 2005).

- Body parts can store highly emotional and traumatic experiences and become implicit memories which then affect movement and behaviour (Schwartz 1980; Rothschild 2000).
- Higher rates of fetal morbidity associated with abnormal labour and dystocia (Saunders et al 2006).
- Mental health in childhood and throughout life negatively affected by birth interventions and analgesia (Jacobsen et al 1987; Raine et al 1997).
- Biological functions of newborn babies may be adversely affected by reduced colostral beta endorphin galactopoiesis in distressed mothers (Zanardo et al 2001).

As has been demonstrated, severe and chronic maternal stress hormones, peptides and immune cells disrupt and dysregulate the unborn baby's nervous system networks affecting regulatory and neurotransmitter systems. These disturbances would include enteric nervous system wiring and functioning. I suggest that irritable bowel syndrome, colic and other digestive system ailments have their genesis in pregnancy too.

UNWANTED BABIES

Being unwanted creates one of the most toxic environments and damaging experiences for unborn babies. The psychological literature has numerous accounts of negative conception memories and the way they have influenced people's lives (Schwarz 1980; Speyrer 1995; Chamberlain 1998; Rothschild 2000; Verny and Weintraub 2002). Dramatic examples of how the dynamics around conception influence the lives of babies and children are found in studies involving unwanted babies. Unwanted babies are at risk on every level of human development. If they make it through to viability, they are more likely to:

- be born prematurely (White 1990; Safanova and Leparski 1998; Orr et al 2000; Wadhwa et al 2001);
- be stillborn (Sable et al 1997);
- be bottle fed (D'Angelo et al 2004);
- develop psychosocial difficulties (Watter 1980);
- have stunted growth (Shapiro-Mendoza et al 2005);
- demonstrate poor and deteriorating school performance (Baydar 1995);
- be exposed to family violence (Gramararian et al 1995);
- have mothers who continued to smoke (Hellerstedt et al 1998);
- have mothers who drink alcohol (Alati et al 2006) with the attendant consequences of those behaviours.

For reasons that are not yet understood, unwanted boys are more likely to suffer these outcomes than unwanted girls (David and Matejcek 1981).

The organ or process affected by maternal stress hormones, toxins or malnutrition depends on the stage of development and gestation when these disruptions occur. It also depends on the individual's genetic inheritance and susceptibility. Severity and longevity of maternal distress state is another key aspect in how stress affects the unborn baby's development. Early programming affects metabolic 'set' points that define the adaptive allostatic range of the individual's physiological activity. These set points may limit or constrain adaptability and so influence susceptibility to diseases such as cardiac disease, hypertension and diabetes in later life. For example, fetal heart rates were significantly raised and stayed higher longer in babies of chronically stressed expectant women who had high levels of stress hormones compared with babies of women with wanted pregnancies, good self-esteem and sufficient social support and low levels of stress hormones. These latter women had calm babies whose heart rate returned to normal quickly. Pregnancy specific anxieties, such as fear of problems with the health and integrity of the unborn baby and fear of pain in labour and birth were found to exert the strongest negative effect on infant development and behaviour (Mulder et al 2002).

The problem is that most women are unaware that their thinking (spiritual focus) and emotional response to life events and circumstances has huge implications for their developing babies. I certainly didn't know. I understood the importance of nutrition, drugs, exercise and rest but I was totally unaware that my spiritual and emotional expression could impact my baby in either negative or positive ways.

IMAGINING HEALTHY BABIES AND NORMAL BIRTHS – A SPIRITUAL PRACTICE AND QUANTUM PROCESS

Australian Aboriginal people are well known for their dreamtime accounts about the origin and formation of the physical world. They dream the future by 'throwing the road out ahead and dreaming it up' (Watson 1999). Day dreaming and imagining the future is now understood to be an important attribute of human brains and nervous systems (Wilkinson 2006). Activating

neural networks by consciously invoking the imagination provides a means by which people can think about their lives, what they want and how they want to be. For women and their partners, the capacity to imagine themselves as parents is part of spiritual preparation for parenthood. The capacity to consciously imagine or visualize the future you desire is one of many quantum processes. Called 'visualization', it is the conscious use of imagination with all senses involved and is an effective way of preparing for future events. Sports psychologists know this brain capacity well and help athletes become winners by encouraging them to imagine winning as part of their preparation. Neural networks of the brain associated with particular body movements fire as if the body actually moved when a person imagines making those movements (Ehrsson et al 2003). The person's physiological state changes as messenger molecules are released in response to the visualization. Physiology follows the conscious mind. In the same way that sportspeople can guide these processes consciously, so too can parents consciously connect with their baby and imagine themselves having a normal birth with a happy, healthy baby breastfeeding beautifully. This establishes a healthy, happy physiology for optimal gene expression and baby materialization.

 To encourage spiritual and emotional development of intending parents, midwives can:
- Point out to parents-to-be the importance of thinking about and emotionally connecting with their developing baby.
- Help parents-to-be develop and explore their ideas and feelings about birth and parenting.
- Help them to imagine:
  - how they want to give birth
  - how they want to feed their baby
  - what kind of parents they want to be
  - what these changes mean for their lives.

The richness of the mother's emotional life not only primes the baby's regulatory and subconscious physiological processes and behaviour, it also lays down the foundations of the baby's implicit memory and personality (Perry et al 1995).

THE POWER AND INFLUENCE
OF PRENATAL BIRTH MEMORIES

Difficult as it is to accept, everyone has implicit memories of their intrauterine, birth and infant experiences (Grof 1985; Chamberlain 1998; Mauger 2000). These memories are, for the most part, subconscious and preverbal and therefore not available to the conscious mind on a day-to-day basis. Implicit memories are expressed as body memories, habits, emotional responses and motor sequence/behaviour (Siegal 1999). An interesting example of an implicit birth memory becoming explicit occurred when I attended a seminar in March 2006, at Darling Harbour in Sydney. After a Neuro-Linguistic Programming (NLP) process on limiting beliefs, a young man, who I will call Mark, stood up and shared his experience of that exercise. I spoke to Mark at the lunch-break and he agreed to let me quote his story as it is an excellent example of how implicit prenatal memories have long term effects on our lives and experiences.

As Mark's story indicates, birth provides a profound emotional experience for the baby and the mother with lifelong consequences. Emotions generated during birth provide an opportunity

for both mother and baby to further accelerate their attachment and deepen their relationship. Please see Chapters 5 and 7 for more details on the hormonal cascades of the love hormone, oxytocin at birth. As the baby grows into a child and later an adult, the prenatal and birth related patterns will underpin his/her worldview and subsequent habitual patterns of response.

MIDWIVES: SETTING THE TRAJECTORY OF HUMAN DESTINY

The act of holding and being held, skin to skin, smelling, touching, feeling, breastfeeding and making eye contact with each other in the first few moments after birth completes reticular formation development in the baby and activates limbic areas in the mother which are responsible for maternal intuition and bonding (Lipton 2005). This bonding is vulnerable in our culture. Mark was born when it was routine to separate mothers and babies at birth. He missed out on the reassuring, emotionally enriching experience of skin to skin experience with his mother at birth. Instead, like the majority of people in our Western culture, he was taken to the nursery to be handled by strangers and left abandoned to cry in isolation. Such treatment is devastating for a newborn and its sense of self (Prescott 1969; Schore 2002). When mother–baby attachment is ruptured and not mended, it leads to violence in the offspring (Prescott 1969; Raine, Brennan and Mednick 1997).

Mark's story

'In this exercise I chose to address the limiting belief that I was unworthy. I felt like this all my life. I always found everything a very real struggle. I felt I had to work harder than everyone else to justify my existence. Everything I have achieved has been through very hard perseverance and it was like I was unworthy to have anything easily or just be happy and relaxed. As we followed instructions to close our eyes and think back to the very first time we felt unworthy, I had no idea what I would recall. I half expected some religious indoctrination scene, however, I suddenly saw and felt myself in my birth.

Immediately I could see and sense the overwhelming level of pain and anguish that my mother, the person I loved more than anything in the world, was experiencing. Tears flowed as I felt overcome with the guilt I felt at my birth. I had at that point during my birth, decided I was unworthy to have anything good or easy in my life. This belief, that I was guilty and it was my fault that she suffered, has impacted on every area of my life.'

 It is a midwife's responsibility to promote the most advantageous development of the infant's reticular formation, emotional, biobehavioural regulatory systems, and facilitate optimal attachment between mothers and their newborns. Midwives are agents of social harmony or disharmony in the way they act at birth. To promote social harmony, they must do everything in their power to provide an environment for the birthing woman and baby in which their relationship can flourish. Midwives must actively change childbirth practices which disrupt infant brain development and mother baby relationships.

As birth is such an emotional time and emotions are memory fixatives, fusing bio-behavioural states into neural networks (Siegal 1999), the effects of unsatisfactory prenatal conditions can, to some extent, be reversed by sensitive supportive care of the birthing mother and the mother baby relationship. One of the most critically important ways of providing sensitive supportive care for birthing women and their babies is through facilitating undisturbed skin to skin time with each other at birth. A study by De Chateau and Wiberg (1984) showed that mothers given extra skin-to-skin time with their babies in the first hour after birth were more responsive to their babies at the three months follow up. These mothers looked face-to-face more often and spent more time kissing their babies than the control group. In addition these infants smiled more often and cried less frequently. One year later, the skin-to-skin mothers held and touched their infants more frequently, talked positively to their infants and stayed at home with their babies longer before returning to professional employment than routine care mothers. More extra contact babies slept in their own rooms, including babies of those mothers in the extra contract group who had returned to work, than the control group. Extra contact babies were ahead of the control group on a developmental schedule. The skin-to-skin mothers breastfed their babies for 2½ months longer than the control group. Videos of interactions between mothers and babies in the skin-to-skin extended contact group showed they laughed more often and talked about and solved differences of opinion more often than control group (De Chateau and Wiberg 1984). The rich sensory stimulation of the newborn baby from the sight (Breiter et al 1996) touch, taste, smell and movement of the mother's body at birth, and during the breastfeeding relationship, wires in the somatosensory and vestibular limbic associative areas of the brain. In this way the neuroassociative brain is mapped with the gestalt of love, trust, intimacy and affection, which subsequently influences the development of later sexual affectional behaviours and wellbeing of the individual (Prescott 1969; Bartels and Zeki 2004).

CONCLUSION

Billions of health dollars are being poured into changing people's brains and bodies once mental, emotional and physical health deficits have become apparent. Although these health deficits usually appear later in life, they are increasingly being recognized as having their genesis in the pre and perinatal period. Using major interventions to treat disease caused by suboptimal pre and perinatal environments is like 'closing the gate after the horse has bolted'. We can be far more effective with our health dollar. The process of building healthy brains and bodies begins before gene transcription and genomic imprinting and requires the most advantageous environment. Heredity is important, but the right environment is equally crucial to healthy development.

Some women enjoy an environment with many aspects that match the most advantageous personal and social situation for childbearing. Some women are able to get their spiritual and emotional needs met. The sad truth is that most don't. Science is providing clear reasons for putting healthy, happy, supported motherhood and by extension fatherhood, at the heart of social and health policy. Maternity services have a duty of care to provide an environment in which women are helped to get their needs met. Midwives have a central role in supporting childbearing women holistically, not only physically, but also emotionally and spiritually. With such care, people's brains and bodies have more chance of being built well from the beginning of life, saving a great deal of individual and societal misery, heartache, disability and ill health.

Insights that I describe within this chapter provide a rich field for further research. They offer compelling evidence for relationship based midwifery care and effective, holistic and practical support for women and their partners/families throughout their childbearing experience. This chapter argues for maternity services to shift their focus from an industrial model to a social, primary health care model. Such a shift is essential because when the mother feels loved, listened to, in control and cared for, her physiology works well and her baby has the best chance of developing normally. The scientific shift in perspective from the Newtonian view of a mechanical material universe to a Quantum physics perspective of an interconnected field of possibilities provides the information and tools to assist with that social and cultural transformation. My challenge to you is to use this information to create the most advantageous spiritual, emotional and physical environment for all mothers, babies and families. The future of our species depends on it.

References

Alati RAL, Mamum A, Williams G, O'Callaghan M, Najman J, Bor W 2006 In utero alcohol exposure and prediction of alcohol disorders in early adulthood. Archives of General Psychiatry 63(9): 1009–1016.

Austin MP, Leader LR, Reilly N 2005 Prenatal stress, the hypothalamic–pituitary–adrenal axis, and fetal and infant neurobehaviour. Early Human Development 81(11): 917–926.

Barker DJP 1998 Mothers, babies and health in later life, 2nd edn. Churchill Livingstone, Edinburgh.

Bartels A and Zeki S 2004 The neural correlates of maternal and romantic love. Neuroimage 21(3): 1155–1166.

Baydar N 1995 Consequences for children of their birth planning status. Family Planning Perspectives 27(6): 228–234.

Beversdorf DQ, Manning SE, Hillier A et al 2005 Timing of prenatal stressors and autism journal of autism and developmental disorders 35(4): 471–478.

Breiter HC, Etcoff NL, Whalen PJ et al 1996 Response and habituation of the human amygdala during visual processing of facial expression neuron. 17(5): 875–887.

Carlson NR 2004 Physiology of behaviour, 8th edn. Pearson Education, Boston.

Chamberlain D 1998 The mind of your newborn baby, 1st edn. North Atlantic Books, Berkeley.

Chilton Pearce J 2004 Nurturance: Integral health and healing. Shift: At the Frontiers of Consciousness. Institute of Noetic Sciences. June August: 16–19.

David HP, Matejcek Z 1981 Children born to women denied abortion: An update Family Planning Perspectives 13(1): 32–34.

D'Angelo DV, Gilbert BC, Rochat RW, Santelli JS, Herold JM 2004 Differences between mistimed and unwanted pregnancies among women who have live births. Perspectives on Sexual and Reproductive Health 36(5): 192–197.

de Chateau P, Wiberg B 1984 Long-term effect on mother–infant behaviour of extra contact during the first hour postpartum. Follow up at one year. Scandanavian Journal of Society and Medicine 12(2): 91–103.

de Kloet ER, Siburg R, Helmerhorst FM, Schmidt M 2005 Stress, genes and the mechanism of programming the brain for later life. Neuroscience and Biobehavioral Reviews 29(2): 271–281.

Ehrsson HH, Geyer S, Naito E 2003 Imagery of voluntary movement of fingers, toes and tongue activates corresponding body part specific motor representations. Journal of Neurophysiology 90(5): 3304–3316.

England MA 1996 Life before birth, 2nd edn. Mosby-Wolfe, Ipswich.

Gershon M 1999 The second brain: A groundbreaking new understanding of nervous disorders of the stomach and intestine. HarperCollins, New York.

Goleman D 1996 Emotional intelligence, 1st edn. Bloomsbury Publishing, London.

Gramararian JA, Adams MM, Saltzman LE et al 1995 The relationship between pregnancy intendedness and physical violence in mothers of newborns. The PRAMS Working Group. Obstetrics and Gynaecology 85(6): 1031–1038.

Grof S 1985 Beyond the brain. New York State University Press.

Hansen D, Lou HC, Olsen J 2000 Serious life events and congenital malformations: A national study with complete follow up. Lancet 356: 875–880.

Heartmath 2002 The inside story, understanding the power of feelings. The Institute of Heartmath, Boulder.

Hellerstedt WL, Pirie PL, Lando HA et al 1998 Differences in preconceptual and prenatal behaviours in women with intended and unintended pregnancies. American Journal of Public Health 88(4): 663–666.

Herlenius E, Lagercrantz H 2004 Development of neurotransmitter systems during critical periods. Experimental Neurology 190(1): 8–21.

Heron J 1989 The facilitator's handbook. Kogan Page, London.

Huizink AC, Mulder EJH, Buitelaar JK 2004 Prenatal stress and risk for psychopathology: Specific effects or induction of general susceptibility? Psychological Bulletin 130(1): 115–142.

Jacobson B, Eklund G, Hamberger L, Linnarsson D, Sedvall G, Velverius M 1987 Perinatal origin of adult self destructive behaviour. Acta Psychiatric Scandinavia 76(4): 364–371.

Lemaire V, Koehl M, Moal ML, Abrous DN 2000 Prenatal stress produces learning deficits associated with an inhibition of neurogenesis in the hippocampus. Neurobiology 97(20):11032–11037.

Lichtarowicz A 2003 Infertility linked to 9/11/ stress Retrieved 16/10/2003 from http://newsvote.bbc.co.uk/mpapps/pagetools/print/news/bbc.co.uk/l/hi/health/3192836.stm.

Lipton BH 2005 The biology of belief. Santa Rosa Mountain of Love/Elite Books.

Mastorakos G, Paviatou MG, Mizamtsidi M 2006 The hypothalamic–pituitary–adrenal and the hypothalamic–pituitary–gonadal axes interplay. Pediatric Endocrinology Review 3 (Supplement 1): 172–181.

Matthews SG 2002 Early programming of the hypothalamo–pituitary–adrenal axis. Trends in Endocrinology and Metabolism 13(9): 73–380.

Mauger B 2000 Reclaiming the spirituality of birth, 1st edn. Rochester Healing Arts Press.

Mulder EJH, Medina PGR, Huizink AC et al 2002 Prenatal maternal stress: Effects on pregnancy and the (unborn) child. Early Human Development 70(1–2): 3–14.

Nepomnacshy PA, Welch KB, McConnell DS et al 2006 Cortisol levels and very early pregnancy loss. Proceedings of the National Academy of Science USA 103(10): 3938–3942.

O'Connor TG, Ben-Shlomo Y, Heron J, Golding J, Adams D, Glover V 2005 Prenatal anxiety predicts individual differences in cortisol in pre-adolescent. Children Biological Psychiatry 58(3): 211–217.

O'Louglin E 2006 8/7/06 Sonic boom attacks spread trauma across Gaza. Sydney Morning Herald: 1.

Orr ST, Miller CA, James SA, Babones S 2000 Unintended pregnancy and preterm birth. Paediatric and Perinatal Epidemiology 14(4): 309–313.

Panksepp J 2001 The long-term psychobiological consequences of infant emotions: Prescriptions for the 21st century. Infant Mental Health Journal 22(1): 132–173.

Perry B Pollard R Blakely T William L and Vigilante D 1995 Childhood trauma, the neurobiology of adaption and use dependant development of the brain: How states become traits. Infant Mental Health Journal 16(4): 271–291.

Pert C 1997 Molecules of emotion: The science behind mind–body medicine. Scribner, New York.

Peterson G 1981 Birthing normally mindbody. Berkeley Press.

Porges SW, Doussard-Roosevelt JA, Stifter CA et al 1999 Sleep state and vagal regulation of heart period patterns in the human newborn: An extension of the polyvagal theory. Psychophysiology 36: 14–21.

Power ML, Schulkin J (Eds) 2005 Birth, distress and disease, 1st edn. Cambridge University Press.

Power ML, Tardiff SD 2005 Maternal nutrition and metabolic control of pregnancy. In: M Power (Ed). Birth, distress and disease. Cambridge University Press.

Prescott JW 1969 Early somatosensory deprivation as an ontological process in the abnormal development of the brain and behaviour. Paper presented at the Medical Primatology Conference, New York.

Raine A, Brennan P, Mednick SA 1997 Interaction between birth complications and early maternal rejection in predisposing individuals to adult violence; specificity to serious, early-onset violence. American Journal of Psychiatry 154: 1265–1267.

Rose S 2006 The 21st century brain: Explaining, mending and manipulating the mind, 1st edn. Jonathon Cape, London.

Rossi EL 2002 The psychobiology of gene expression, 1st edn. WW Norton, London.

Rothschild B 2000 The body remembers, 1st edn. New York WW Norton and Company Inc.

Sable MR, Spencer JC, Stockbauer JW et al 1997 Pregnancy wantedness and adverse pregnancy outcomes: Differences by race and Medicaid status. Family Planning Perspectives 29(2): 76–81.

Safonova T, Leparksy EA 1998 The unwanted child: Child abuse and negligence. 22(2): 155–157.

Saunders TA, Lobel M, Veloso C, Meyer B 2006 Prenatal maternal stress is associated with delivery analgesia and unplanned caesareans. Journal of Psychosomatic Obstetrics: 1–6.

Schore AN 2002 The neurobiology of attachment and early personality organization. Journal of Prenatal and Perinatal Psychology and Health (16).

Schulkin J, Schmidt L, Erikson K 2005 Glucocorticoid facilitation of corticotrophin-releasing-hormone in the placenta and the brain: Functional impact on behavior. In: J Schulkin, ML Power (Eds). Birth, distress and disease, 1st edn, pp. 235–267, Cambridge University Press.

Schwartz L 1980 The world of the unborn, 1st edn. Richard Marek, New York.

Shapiro-Mendoza C, Selwyn BJ, Smith DP, Sanderson M 2005 Parental pregnancy intention and early childhood stunting: findings from Bolivia. International Journal of Epidemiology 34(2): 387–396.

Siegal DJ 1999 The developing mind, 1st edn. The Guilford Press, New York.

Sugiura-Ogasawara M, Furukawa TA, NakanoY et al 2002 Depression as a potential causal factor in subsequent miscarriage in recurrent spontaneous aborters. Human Reproduction 17(10): 2580–2584.

Speyrer JA 1995 The primal psychotherapy. Page retrieved 24/10/06, from http://primal-page.com/index.html

Tsiaras A 2002 From conception to birth. Random House, Sydney.

Teixeira JMA, Fisk NM, Glover V 1999 Association between maternal anxiety in pregnancy and increased uterine artery resistance index: Cohort based study. British Medical Journal 318(7177): 53–157.

Uvnas-Moberg K 2003 The oxytocin factor: Tapping the hormone of calm, love and healing. Da Capo, Cambridge.

Uvnas-Moberg K, Arn I, Magnusson D 2005 The psychobiology of emotion: The role of the oxytocinergic system. International Journal of Behavioral Medicine 12: 59–65.

Van den Bergh B, Mennes M, Oosterlaan J et al 2005 High antenatal maternal anxiety is related to impulsivity during performance on cognitive tasks in 14 and 15 year olds. Neuroscience and Biobehavioral Reviews 29(2): 259–269.

Van Den Bergh BRH, Mulder EJH, Mennes M, Glover V 2005 Antenatal maternal anxiety and stress and the neurobehavioural development of the fetus and child: Links and possible mechanisms. Neuroscience and Biobehavioral Reviews 29(2): 237–258.

Verny T, Weintraub P 2002 Tomorrow's baby, 1st edn. Simon and Schuster, New York.

Wadhwa PD 2005 Psychoneuroendocrine processes in human pregnancy influence fetal development and health. Psychoneuroendocrinology 30(8): 724–743.

Wadhwa PD, Sandman CA, Garite TJ 2001 The neurobiology of stress in human pregnancy: Implications for prematurity and development of the fetal central nervous system. Progress in Brain Research 133: 131–142.

Watter WW 1980 Mental Health Consequences of abortion and refused abortion. Canadian Journal of Psychiatry 25(1): 68–73.

Watson J 1999 Postmodern nursing and beyond. Churchill Livingstone, London.

Weinstock M 2005 The potential influence of maternal stress hormones on development and mental health of the offspring. Brain, Behavior and Immunity 9(4): 296–308.

Welberg LAM, Secki JR 2001 Prenatal stress, glucocorticoids and the programming of the brain. Journal of Neuroendocrinology 13(2): 113.

White AE 1990 The incidence of unplanned and unwanted pregnancies among live births from health visitor records. Child Care and Health Development 16(4): 219–226.

Wilkoinson M 2006 The dreaming mind–brain: A Jungian perspective. Journal of Analytical Psychology 51(1): 43–59.

Yoles IMH, Kaplan B, Ovadia J 1993 Fetal 'fright bradycardia' brought on by air-raid alarm in Israel. International Journal of Gynaecology and Obstetrics 40(2): 157–160.

Zanardo V, Nicolussi S, Favaro F et al 2001 Effect of postpartum anxiety on the colostrol milk g-endorphin concentrations of breastfeeding mothers. Journal of Obstetrics and Gynaecology 21(2): 130–134.

Chapter 7

Mindbodyspirit architecture: Creating birth space

Bianca Lepori
Maralyn Foureur
Carolyn Hastie

'Years ago at a dinner party with a group of fellow architects, I was asked for my view of the City of London master-plan and whether I thought it should have been altered in any way. My reply was that (in those days) I was primarily concerned with one room only; the first room we enter when we come into this world. I will never forget the pitiful glance my answer received – or my companion's farewell words at the end of the evening. "I look forward to hearing more about your work when you grow up!" Because of my role as an architect, I was and I am supposed to have ideas about how space should be organized. The bigger the space I can organize, the bigger architect I am. Therefore it seemed to my dinner companion that there was no point in concentrating on one room, particularly on such an obvious one – a room whose layout had already been set up and seemed to work quite effectively all over the world. Why not simply repeat it endlessly and get on with real architecture?' (Bianca Lepori)

INTRODUCTION: BIANCA LEPORI

What is real architecture, one may ask? Can architecture get away without posing fundamental questions based on philosophical, physiological and humanistic issues; without understanding how to shape and reshape spaces drawing inspiration from people and their creativity? The intention here is to share how, starting from the birthing room, awareness has been brought to my architectural practice in general as well as to the way birthing rooms are designed. The image of the modern birth space is of a large, tiled and bright room; blinding white light; chromium plated equipment surrounding a small, tall, narrow bed standing right in the middle of the room and even perhaps facing a door kept open onto the passage way. In institutional labour rooms around the developed world it is plain to see that most women lie down to give birth on their backs. In many places it is still possible to see women with their legs lifted up in the air and tied to hangers in order to give birth. The women are passive objects and the birth attendants are the special subjects of the scene, performing specialized roles. This is an image that belongs to the age of modernity; the machine age where birth came to be seen as not a normal function of human beings, but a process that has to be kept under control, because it is potentially pathological.

How do we feel in these places and spaces? Do they welcome us and listen to us? Can we feel comfortable, move and express ourselves at ease? Women who do not accept this way of birth have to fight against an attitude which keeps proposing the horizontal position as the only admissible way of coming into the world. This imposed position is only made possible because women are forced to adjust themselves to environments made up of impersonal spaces, impersonal actions and psychological constraints. Although the possibility of surgical birth has removed the risk of death or injury for those women and babies who have developed some pathological condition, making space to accommodate the potential for a surgical birth has irrevocably changed the process for healthy mothers and babies too. I am reminded of the words of Elias Canetti who said '...the most dangerous thing about technology is that it makes us forget what man really is [and] what he really needs' (Canetti 1983).

We need not take this image for granted. It is not the only, nor indeed a necessary way to create a birth space. Birth spaces designed for 'housing' the psycho-physical expressiveness of the woman and child, and the emotive and affective expressiveness of the family require a radical shift built on an understanding that physical spaces are not only our spatial environments but also places of the soul within us. A radical new birth architecture will put advanced technology to man's service in a human way to integrate the whole map of biology, engineering and religion to substitute the antagonism of the left and right hemispheres of the brain leading to an integration and 'best of both worlds' view.

We have called this chapter 'Mindbodyspirit Architecture: Creating Birth Space' to emphasize the importance of an understanding of mindbodyspirit even in the building of the physical location for birth, in order for birth to occur optimally. The theories and understanding that have motivated and supported my learning and practice in architecture are joined in the second half of this chapter, by the learning and practice of two midwifery colleagues to explore the possibilities for creating birth spaces that enable women to labour and give birth without disruption to the healthy dynamic flow of mother and baby neuro-physiology.

PART 1

THE MOVING, FEELING AND DREAMING BODY GUIDES ARCHITECTURAL DESIGN: BIANCA LEPORI

Any engagement with a design process requires a starting point of innocence. The architect must be oblivious to the status quo and must develop clarity about who the actors and acted-upon subjects of the scene are. This is because any subjects experience space with at least three bodies: *the moving, the feeling* and *the dreaming body* and all three are affected by design and thus deserve concern along with any design process (Franck and Lepori 2007). We will return to this concept often throughout the chapter. The second lesson is that pathways, as the structure of the speech of architecture, become the key element of a rigorous design. They give order or disorder to space, whose distribution cannot be accidental or arbitrary, even in the most spontaneous of settings. As in nature, where spontaneity, beauty and even wilderness are based on mathematics, space is based on underlying patterns of organization. It is through the arrangement of partitions or other types of barriers, such as furniture or even low walls, that people are led along a sequence of spaces with different sizes, proportions, orientation, colour and texture; each becoming a sentence contributing to the story of a particular place (Franck and Lepori 2007).

A room, like the typical birthing room in an institutional setting, cannot be limited by formulae to be simply a technologically aware layout dictated by packages of functionality defined to meet business needs. To structure such a room from the point of view of *all* its users rather than only with technology and standards in mind, may increase its efficiency. Considering the needs of all its users may also define appropriateness to its functions and the need to interrelate with other systems. This will enable us to move away from spaces designed as fleshless skeletons, whose arrow-like pathways indicate, one by one, the steps that lead to a successful outcome – without taking into account people's *moving, feeling and dreaming bodies*.

Moving from home to hospital shifts the focus from physiology to pathology

It was only after the second post-war period that the concept of birth as a natural event was replaced by a concept connected to the hospital and medical environment. Until then women never thought of having to or being able to leave their homes to give birth to their children. It was natural for them, their husbands and their relatives to identify the birth scene with their home environment, as much as today the delivery scene is usually identified with the hospital.

For the first time in human history the science of gynaecology has enabled us to know and see (to a certain extent) what goes on inside a woman's body during her pregnancy. This has allowed us to look into, follow and check the biological mystery, and provide some answers for when birth is difficult. Women and men have been reassured by the science of pathological birth and have come to realize that the new medical–technological options for birth are also a way to entrust others with the burden and responsibility of an inescapable, and often only painfully suffered, fate. Therefore many women actively or unconsciously chose to give up the hard work involved in consciously participating in the event and handed over control to others. The result is that women assumed a passive role in childbirth and physiological childbirth all but disappeared. From a design perspective the focus shifted from the woman and baby and their needs to the needs of the medical technologists who became the major actors in the space.

The space generated by the hospital logic is serially arranged with simplified straight paths which point out the promptness operators are bound to comply with. The hierarchy is imposed by a theoretic pathway, which implicitly delegates the responsibility of birth to specialized people invested with a specific authority to perform specialized and routine interventions. The pathways of a hospital birthing room are 'planned on paper' according to a pathological view of birth which sees a narrow tall bed as the focus of the room. The bed is identified as the only piece of furniture the woman can use, possibly surrounded by people standing around her. Although it ignores the 'individual interior pathways' meant to help most women to identify their own territory of comfort, this model is assumed to be the only one needed for all births.

New techniques and technology are capable of preventing and avoiding most risks and complications which, according to data collected by the World Health Organization, concern no more than 20% of women in childbirth. As a consequence, 80% of births are normal, proving that the ideal scientific 'one size fits all' model for childbirth and birthplaces seems to be not only inadequate but irrational for most births that do not need to be performed according to a monitored protocol.

To explore another pathway to counterbalance the status quo model for birth space may allow women to re-connect with being present and actively participating in the event. To complement the space/model, the technologic–scientific one, characterized by functionality, bright light and linearity, it is necessary to design a space/way which is psychobiological, functional to the dynamics of birth as an event belonging to the sexual and sensitive sphere. Such a space/way will have to offer freedom as well as logic, be capable of accepting disorder, of being a place of gestalt synthesis, of holding the continuity of the event according to its stages and natural rhythms. It will have to suit both categories of subjects – operators and women as well as being motivated by and adapted to the functions of both hemispheres of the brain.

The concept of childbirth, as an event or an intervention respectively lived at home or in hospital, may be viewed as connected both to the right or the left hemisphere of the brain. The former houses the archaic image of women's idols, typical of matriarchal societies where the woman, as the earth, is prolific and nourishes. The latter, equivalent to the sphere of consciousness, contains the cognitive capacity and rational logic which enables people to analyse and attempt to control the ambivalence of nature itself.

The functional characteristics of the brain hemispheres can be summarized as in Box 7.1, or as visual symbols, as in Figure 7.1.

In designing birth places the exercise might be to create spaces based on a specific relationship between the two opposite poles: the hospital inspired by a left hemisphere, technological approach, and a home space, primarily based on the right hemisphere of the everyday, domestic life. This way the spaces for birth can safeguard

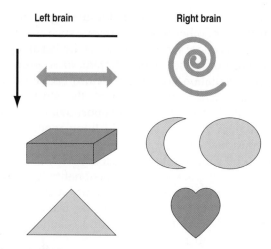

Figure 7.1   Visual representation of left brain and right brain functions.

analytical layouts with a touch of attention and care for women's needs and become more women and children aware.

The symbols of home – metaphysical spaces

In order to revisit birth places with women in mind and find out what technology has made us forget, it is important to analyse how women give birth in their own territory, at home. Home, the symbolic place which reproduces in each of us the feeling of the prenatal period when our entire psychophysical system was protected by a soft and round inside, is a dress which fits us perfectly, as the original womb, the enveloping and padded pocket which nourishes us while moulding itself according to our growth during the time we spend alone in the dim light. Home is of feminine gender; it is an interior space as well as boundary to our personal expression. The values, pathways and movements of women choosing their own homes to give birth can provide important insights into qualitative models, which may be used to integrate current medical care. The following stories were derived from interviews with women in Modena, Italy. Both the women who preferred their homes to the hospital and those who were 'confined' to their domestic space because of the lack of hospital care in the area, tell of the simple physical pathway that on approaching labour,

Box 7.1 The functional characteristics of the brain hemispheres (Lepori 1992)	
Left hemisphere	**Right hemisphere**
Verbal	Visual-spatial
Logical	Synthetic
Analytical	Intuitive
Sequential	Simultaneous
Direct	Free
Rational	Mythical
Critical	Existential
Abstract	Map-like
Differential	Holistic
Digital	Analogical
Planned	Spontaneous
Quantitative	Qualitative

helped them to find themselves, in a limited environment – an individual territory, similar to the territory that the females of other mammals instinctively delimit for themselves. Animal similes are used with the women's stories to illustrate the female need to create an individually significant, comfortable, satisfying and safe place for birth.

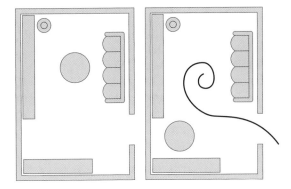

Figure 7.2 Schematic representation of Valeria's room.

Valeria, a she-wolf

The pregnancy of a she-wolf lasts about nine weeks... childbirth usually takes place inside a hole dug in the soft soil by the same animal, or among brambles, which we may call a sort of bed, or sheltered by a rock, or among roots...

The moving of the table has allowed space for movements; the space is both empty and limited by the corner framed by two walls and the carpet where childbirth spontaneously finds its nest and centre (Fig. 7.2).

Tiziana: the she-coyote

A few weeks before delivery, the she-coyote works hard at setting up several dens, which may be even a dozen; only at the last minute she chooses one of these...

The place chosen for delivery varies according to the women's nature as their movements vary during childbirth. Some women keep still on all fours or crouch. Some others feel like walking. The bed then becomes the pallet-nest – the small room – the den.

Valeria's story

'I moved out of my previous home in May and gave birth to my child at the end of July, thus the new place did not feel like home to me. The only room I really felt comfortable in, because I had arranged it myself (I had hung all my pictures and set the bookshelves in order) was the dining room which was the most pleasant room where I also used to spend plenty of time with my friends. On approaching labour, I moved away the small table in front of the couch and covered the floor with a carpet. During labour, I was on all fours. I also used the couch (which is very large) in different ways to lean on, when I didn't lean on my husband. When the head started to come out, he sat on the couch and my child came to the world while I was crouching on the carpet, held between my husband's knees.'

Tiziania's story

'We live on the fourth floor, an apartment made up of a living room, a kitchen, a bathroom and a bedroom. It's a place I've never liked. I started loving it when I was three or four months pregnant. I badly needed to build a nest: I felt a desire for a home as I never did before. Until that morning I didn't know where birth would take place. At home or at the hospital? I could not work out where I would find most support. Then, when the first slight pains started, I realized that I wanted to be in a very private place, made up of small, limited and poorly lit spaces.

Until that moment I'd thought that childbirth could have taken place in the living room, because I was used to spending a long time sitting on the couch. That morning, when the first pains started, though, I was tidying up the bedroom and there I stayed. I remember starting to walk in that room, back and forth; the furniture there consisted of a large bed, a wardrobe, and a table. The room was small and I kept walking back and forth. I felt the first push while I was standing up; it felt so strong that I had to counterbalance it by getting down on my hands and knees on the bed where I stayed until Lucia came to the world. Both the bed and the mattress are hard. I gave birth on a corner of the bed. I looked at my husband in front of me; I didn't let him move even if he wanted to see how the baby was coming out. Looking at him gave me strength.'

Alessandra: the female gazelle

A short time before delivery the female gazelle moves away from the herd and carefully chooses a suitable place to give birth into the grass.

The layout of this large space allowed the woman to make a choice and to identify 'sub-zones' delimited by the walls and the furniture. The corner between the wall and the low furniture in this case supplied protection and support to the event.

Fiorella: the female cheetah

The female cheetah gave birth into high grass.

The need for defining a space is a constant; the type of definition varies. What this means is that in preparing for the birth of their infant females of all species have an instinctive urge to define the boundaries and content of the birth place. How this is created is very individual. The two couches within whose 'energy field' the woman finds her centre after moving away the table in this case, represent the high grass. The 'beautiful' painting enhances the sense of belonging to the place; that is the sharing of affection.

These examples show that each woman defines her single-centred territory for labour and birth, where she can concentrate and gather strength. The body always chooses a solid and protected place between furniture and very seldom on it. This centre, not determined by outer authorities or designers or behaviour planners, is defined each time by the action and concentration focusing on it, as if representing the intimacy of a heart-

---

Fiorella's story

'I live in an old, very large apartment made of interconnected rooms. I gave birth in the living room between two couches. The living room is an open space because we have pulled down a wall, and so now it is much larger than it used to be. My choice came naturally: the living room is where I spend most of my time, there are couches, to me it's the most comfortable place. The bedroom is a wasted room, I never use it; and then I would never choose it because the bed is very tall and so very uncomfortable for somebody who wants to give birth in "unusual" positions. It's very tall and not very "pleasant".
My living room is not crowded with furniture even if there's a huge bookcase looming over. There are paintings on the walls. I gave birth facing a beautiful one, a very colourful painting. Colour I really love, all blue hues of the "lapis-lazuli" type. It reminds me of water. After the delivery, I stood up and sat on the edge of the couch.'

---

place whose beating does not undergo any interference. By naturally going in towards this centre of action and concentration, each woman builds a micro-environment/micro-cosmos for herself.

The spiral versus the arrow pathway

The symbol of the spiral, which represents the progressive intensification of the delivery process until it ends in the 'birth point', replaces the arrow-path expression of efficiency. The natural spiral path is leading toward the centre of a woman's concentration and ability to listen, thus towards her own control and choice. Women who can give birth naturally do not need particular colours, or beautiful furniture that reminds them of their homes. They do not need a homey atmosphere so much as a space in which they can express themselves and in which they can move around and change position whenever they wish to. They need a space in which to express themselves, in which to wait; they need the space-time to let it happen. The only thing they really need is not to be forced into a particular position. Even pain dissolves with movement; pain-killers are a consequence of stillness.

Thus it becomes clear what 'domestic' means, in relation to birth environments, for the childbearing

---

Alessandra's story

'That was my third delivery. I had other kids to look after, my day had gone on just as usual. I wasn't sure I would give birth that night. I couldn't really choose the room: two kids were sleeping in their bedroom, and my bedroom is next to theirs. The room I spend more time in is the dining room: it's a very large carpeted room, divided in three zones by flower vases and low furniture one can sit on. I crouched, with my head between my hands, keeping my pelvis higher up, in the mid zone near the low furniture. There was a halogen lamp, other lights were on in the room next door.'

woman. It means freedom of movement, the possibility to choose and control comfort and ease, the possibility of relying on fittings that support bodily needs. It means having the power to choose, no matter what she chooses. Mimicking a cosy home environment doesn't go far enough.

To design from the 'inside out', thus from the needs of the three bodies, the one that moves, the one that feels and the one that dreams will complement design based on the needs for safety, security, protection, as well as the needs of giving up and letting the 'expert' or 'practitioners' handle the management of birth and perform the delivery. Having understood that women who have given birth at home never expose themselves at the centre of the scene such as the prominently placed delivery bed implies; having documented that, when free to follow their natural urges during childbirth, women tend to choose an empty protected area, such as a sitting room, rather than a bedroom. With their feet solidly on the floor, they kneel, crouch and use other postures that relax the pelvic floor and allow gravity to help birth to take place.

The design implications are that we have to eliminate the bed as the central focus of a delivery space. We need the backup of the contemporary medical world, but in more flexible, woman-centred spaces. Beside moving the bed away from the centre of the birthing room, various means of support need to be scattered throughout the room; such as bars women can hold on to; benches at various heights they can lay their elbows on; soft fabric ropes hanging from the ceiling they can grab in order to release pelvic tension; movable birthing stools. Even better than a bed would be a large platform on which a woman could sit, kneel, rest, lie down, stand again or kneel on the floor with her elbows on the platform. Since water can relieve pain and accelerate dilation, a pool makes sense within the delivery space as well.

All theories, forms and suggestions I have proposed are drawn from an experiential approach to design, based on the strong belief that comfortable spaces derive from a careful design, well informed about the needs of its users. It will be obvious that my attitude and mind-set are strongly aligned with midwifery in two ways. The first is in my intent to balance right and left brain functions in design as midwives do in skilled midwifery practice. The second is because the purpose of my work is the same as for a midwife: helping women to give birth to their desires through creating mindbodyspirit birth space.

Towards this aim I will be complemented in the next section of this chapter by my midwifery colleagues (Maralyn Foureur and Carolyn Hastie). Maralyn and Carolyn describe their practice experience of creating and working within environments that enact many of the key design principles I have explored. The next section also examines some theoretical ideas that support the mindbodyspirit design principles and provides a critique of the research that has failed to consider the impact of design elements on birth outcomes, when attempting comparisons of place of birth.

PART 2

PUTTING THE PRINCIPLES INTO PRACTICE: MARALYN FOUREUR AND CAROLYN HASTIE

We first met Bianca a number of years ago when involved in the redesign of the delivery unit of a major maternity hospital in New Zealand. We were thrilled to find an architect who understood at a deeply integrated philosophical, theoretical and physiological level how the physical birth space needed to be constructed in order to provide women with the greatest opportunity to give birth normally. We will examine that redesign process in more detail to follow, but first let's consider whether the design principles that Bianca writes of are only useful in areas where new birth spaces are being designed and built or whether the principles can be applied to the existing maternity units in which most of us work.

For many years (from 1982 onwards) as midwives in private practice in Australia we had supported women to birth in their own homes or in hospitals. The two spaces were worlds apart. At home the woman was free to move as the rhythm of her labour swept her along. We were guests in her space and accommodated ourselves to meet her needs. Women responded in dynamic and dis-inhibited ways to the feeling of the baby pressing on the cervix or moving through the pelvis. Women were quiet and noisy, clothed or naked, restless or still, paced the room, rocked back and forth, sat in chairs, lay on the bed, squatted in the toilet, stood under the shower, lay in the bath, leaned over the mantelpiece or window sill and chose many different locations within their homes in which to give birth; just as in Bianca's stories of women birthing at home in Italy. In the hospital we (midwives and women) found ourselves limited and constrained by the lack of privacy, the lack of accessible bathroom and en-suite facilities, but largely by the only piece of furniture in the room: the high, narrow, metal bed with the plastic undersheet and the ever-ready stirrups. We decided to fold up the bed and push it to the corner of the room; out of the way. Since we encouraged women to bring support people as well as their other children if they wished to share the experience, we were often in the position of having to locate places for them to sit around the edges of the room. Families bought along extra pillows, CD player and CDs of relaxing music, massage oils, food, drinks and ice for the woman to suck, pictures of nature and water, images and things of beauty to rest the eye upon. There were books or games for the children to pass the time as well as their own support person. The room started to get rather crowded. And still the bed exerted its powerful pull.

Against initial opposition from the hospital staff, we eventually decided to remove the bed from the room altogether. We simply wheeled it outside the door. We removed the mattress from the bed and placed it on the floor along with a beanbag and gym mats so that the woman had a choice of places to kneel or squat or lie down during labour and eventually to give birth. We located a very simple birth stool and found that we could modify straight back chairs with pillows and towels to provide sitting and leaning places for the woman. Families bought buckets to fill with hot water and nappies to soak in them to make hotpacks. We turned off the bright overhead lights in the room and turned the large, centrally placed theatre light upwards to face the ceiling where it could provide a gentle suffused light. And we took the clock off the wall. The space gradually took on a more woman friendly look and feel. Eventually we found that the hospital staff would set up the room for us when we called to say we were arriving with a woman in labour. The bed would be outside, the lights turned down low and mats and beanbags in the room. They too had experienced and approved the different mood and the freedom the women were provided by removing the bed from centre stage.

So, in essence we are convinced that *every* birth space can be modified to accommodate the *moving, feeling and dreaming body*. We discovered the principles by comparing the home and hospital birth spaces and by closely observing how women behaved in each place. With the new insights provided by considering the specialization of the left and right brain hemispheres we can now articulate the design principles more clearly as described in Box 7.2.

These principles were enacted in the design and building of what has come to be known as the Lepori Birth Rooms in one maternity unit in New Zealand and the story of how this came about follows.

The construction of the Lepori Birth Rooms

In early 2000, funds were made available at a major maternity hospital to renovate its 1970's birthing unit. One of us (MF) was working there at the time and had by then discovered a journal article written by Bianca called 'Freedom of Movement in Birth Places' (Lepori 1994). We were aware that Bianca was in the southern hemisphere attending a childbirth conference and invited her to come to New Zealand to provide input into the re-design project.

Box 7.2 The moving, feeling and dreaming body

The moving body

Needs: Space and freedom to move; to be able to move to the dance of labour; to respond to the inner movements of the baby; to walk, kneel, stretch, lay down, lean, squat, stand and be still.

The feeling body

Needs: soft and yielding surfaces; or firm and supportive surfaces; to experience different textures; the right temperature; to be touched/or not; to be immersed in water, flowing or still; to feel respected, safe, protected and loved.

The dreaming body

Responds to images, archetypes, colours; responds to soft curves rather than sharp angles; may need to hide in the darkness or dim light; responds to nature.

Needs to remain focused and therefore needs to avoid rational language, harsh sounds, bright lights (these stimulate and distract the neocortex).

Bianca presented her ideas to a specially convened forum of architects, designers, hospital planners, financial manager and medical and midwifery staff of the hospital and found a receptive and open audience. Together with Professor John Gray from Victoria University of Wellington,

Bianca was invited to prepare a sketch of how the space could be modified. The original sketch is included here to illustrate the enactment of the design principles that were developed and the minimal design compromises that had to be made to fit into the available space (Fig. 7.3).

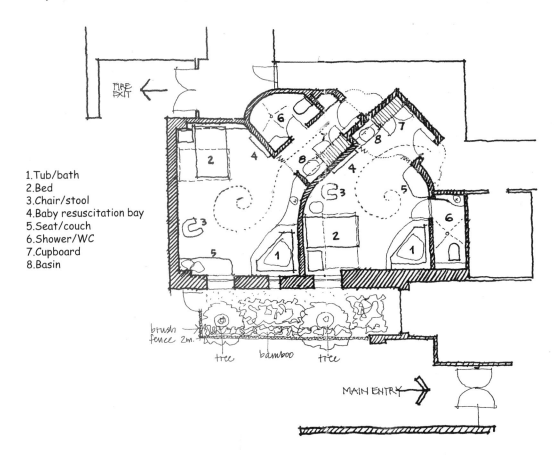

1.Tub/bath
2.Bed
3.Chair/stool
4.Baby resuscitation bay
5.Seat/couch
6.Shower/WC
7.Cupboard
8.Basin

Figure 7.3 Original working sketch for birth rooms, Wellington.

The whole project was presented as one way to address the rising caesarean section rates which were evident in this community. It was proposed that the existing 'production-line' environment with first stage rooms where women laboured and were then transferred to an operating room for the birth of their baby was an extremely stress-filled environment. We were convinced that a new mindbodyspirit birth-space that considered all the sensory modalities involved in the perception of stress or ease would have a positive impact on women's perceptions of anxiety and therefore physiological processes and the progress of labour. The hospital authorities were similarly persuaded to support these concepts and the Lepori Birth Rooms were commissioned.

Box 7.3 contains a summary of the key concepts incorporated in the design of mindbodyspirit birth spaces. Even the colours used in the rooms were deserving of careful consideration to ensure maximum positive impact. By employing an understanding of the body energy system known as chakras (from eastern philosophy/medicine/spirituality), a series of colours that evoke sensory responses in different parts of the body were chosen to cover the walls and for furniture and fittings. Table 7.1 reveals the chakra/colours that may unconsciously assist

---

Box 7.3   Developing mindbodyspirit architecture for birth

Many factors need to be considered in creating optimal birth environments that respect the sacredness of birth.

1. **Female space**
   Feminine archetypes* in artworks: e.g. symbols of goddesses such as Artemis; round, ripe fruits; yin-yang symbol; earth/mother; etc.
   Symbols of beauty, wholeness, harmony
   Cleanliness and order
   Calmness and peacefulness
   Culturally safe

2. **Shapes**
   Soft curves
   Rounded corners and edges to walls and furniture, not right angles

3. **Space**
   Corridor leading to birth room provides protection/privacy/sense of going into a private space
   Location of bed in relation to the door – no direct line of sight
   Door is at the side of the room and is not central
   Empty space of possibilities in the centre of the room
   Low wall for leaning on can protect bed from the doorway
   Pleasant walking space both inside and outside the room
   Medical gases and suction delivery systems need to be provided with long connection tubes and are not centrally located in the room – will be able to be moved where the woman locates herself

4. **Elements of nature**
   Windows onto the outside world are essential
   View of sky, water, mountains, flowers or trees through the window
   Indoor landscaping
   Pictures of nature

5. **Water**
   Bath and shower available
   Bath is part of birth room and not a separate space
   Bath is deep enough so that woman can be totally immersed when on hands and knees
   Two-sided access to the bath
   Bath capacity: wide enough to accommodate the woman comfortably
   Toilet and shower separate to birth room but large enough to give birth in if it occurs there

6. **Texture**
   Textural variety on wall surfaces, floors and ceilings, furniture, fabrics, artworks
   Soft and yielding furnishings
   Firm and strong furniture capable of providing physical support
   Natural materials such as timber, tiles
   Avoid metallic materials in surfaces or trolleys

7. **Privacy**
   Lockable doors – ability to control who enters the room
   Knock before entering
   Respect for personal bodily integrity – ability to control who touches her body and how
   Ethical agreements between women and their carers
   Windows with one-way glass for night privacy so the woman can see out but no-one can see in
   Secure and lockable place for belongings if the woman leaves the room
   Entry door screened so the woman cannot be observed from the doorway
   Moveable screens to hide equipment

8. **Light**
   Natural light through windows or skylights
   Windows low enough to see the view when lying in the bed

Box 7.3 Continued

No overhead lights
Dimmable lighting
No theatre light
Portable extra lighting available

9. Colour
Careful use of colour on walls and furniture and bed linen/towels – see Table 7.1: Chakras/colour

10. Support
Furniture: birth stool, beanbag, gym mat, exercise ball, chairs, bed or platform, extra pillows
Hook in ceiling from which to hang hammock or soft ropes for stretching
Bars on walls at various heights
Mantelpiece or bench for leaning on
Comfortable chair for breastfeeding

11. Noise control
Sound reducing acoustics
CD player for music of woman's choice (not musak)
Sound of footsteps in corridor reduced
Loudspeaker paging system not audible
Staff conversations from 'the desk' or staff lounge not audible
Other women in labour or giving birth in the next room unable to be heard
Clanking of metal instruments on metal trolleys is not heard

12. Thermal comfort
Adjustable to enable woman to be naked at a comfortable temperature
Heating for mother and baby

Blanket warming cupboard

13. Air quality
Aromatherapy oil burner to provide pleasant smell
Fresh air possible through opening windows
Avoidance of odiferous cleaning agents
Avoidance of noxious off-gassing from synthetic materials and medical gases

14. Accommodation for companions and birth attendants
A comfortable place to sit or lay down from time to time
Make companions feel welcome rather than intrusive
Access to vending machines with healthy food and drink options
Access to telephones
Access to cafeteria
Access to toilet and shower
Parking space

15. Food and drink
Available for the woman and her family
Microwave for heating foods
Toaster
Hot water
Refrigerator with ice available

16. Safety
Telephone in the room
Call bell system in the room
Equipment for resuscitation of the mother or baby in cupboards with bi-fold doors or screened
Wet areas must have safety flooring to prevent slipping for woman or staff

*Archetypes are deep enduring patterns of thought and behaviour that are laid down in the human psyche that remain powerful over long periods of time and transcend cultures. Archetypes form the basis of unlearned, instinctual patterns of behaviour that humankind, regardless of culture, shares in common (see also the biophilia hypothesis).

Table 7.1 Chakras/colour and energy spectrum

Chakra	Location	Associated with:-	Colour
First	Base of the spine	Home, security, sense of self Survival, trust	Red
Second	Top of the pubic bone	Sexuality and relationship with other The birthing of something new	Orange
Third	Solar plexus	Ego, power, control, freedom	Yellow
Fourth	Heart	Love, forgiveness and relating	Green
Fifth	Throat	Communication, self expression and receiving information	Blue
Sixth	Middle of forehead	Intuition, insight, wisdom Extra sensory perception (ESP)	Purple
Seventh	Crown of head	Universal consciousness Spirituality	Violet

women to be grounded and in their power for birth.

Many hundreds of women and midwives have used the Lepori Birth Rooms in this setting over the intervening years with many positive comments and positive birth experiences. However, no formal evaluation of the impact of the rooms was undertaken due to an inability to attract research funding. More recently women's views on what they would like to have in the birth space have been sought through a small number of surveys conducted in the UK, Australia and New Zealand (Boulton et al 2003; Foureur 2003; Fraser et al 2003; National Childbirth Trust 2003). It is hardly surprising to find that these same principles are echoed in the women's own words in these surveys.

What do women want in their birth space?

While women's views of the birth experience are often sought, their ideas about the physical, bricks and mortar and furnishings of the birth space have not been well studied. Most satisfaction surveys don't even ask what kind of physical facilities women want or what they need them to contain. Studies have asked women if they would like access to midwifery led or medically led birth units, or whether they prefer home, birth centre or hospitals for birth. None of these studies has described the physical attributes of

each kind of birth space. Studies focus on maternal and neonatal outcomes in different locations and also women's satisfaction measured through responses to components such as personal control and respect, or the model of care (Handler et al 1996; Wiegers et al 1996; Rennie et al 1998; Emslie et al 1999; Kauffman 2000; Coyle et al 2001; Fenwick et al 2004; Walsh and Downe 2004; Hodnett et al 2005; Walsh 2005; Singh and Newburn 2006). It appears that the physical environment for birth is irrelevant.

One exception to this was a magazine and online survey of nearly 2000 women conducted by the National Childbirth Trust in the UK (NCT 2003) to discover if women thought the physical environment had any impact on their birth experience. Nine out of ten women thought the physical surroundings affected how easy or hard it was to give birth. Women listed a range of attributes they thought were very important in the birth environment, but few women actually had access to all the items they thought were very important. Over half of the women *did not have access to any* of these items. Table 7.2 illustrates what women in the NCT study and others have identified is important to them in the physical birth territory.

In addition to control, privacy and physical comfort, the women surveyed emphasized the importance of beauty, nature and ambience in the birth space. Sense sensitive elements such

---

Table 7.2   What women want in the physical birth territory (NCT 2003)

Item	Rating	Source
Clean room with en-suite facilities	High	NCT 2003
Comfortable furniture	High	NCT 2003
Not being watched	High	NCT 2003
Control of heating	High	NCT 2003
Control of lighting	High	NCT 2003
Control of who entered room in labour	High	NCT 2003
Use of birthing pool	High	NCT 2003
Staying in one room	High	NCT 2003 Boulton, Chapple & Saunders 2003
Pillows floor mats and bean bags	High	NCT 2003
Place to get snacks and drinks	High	NCT 2003
Pleasant place to walk	High	NCT 2003
Homely environment	High	NCT 2003 Boulton, Chapple & Saunders 2003 Fraser, Watts & Munir 2003
Soundproof – not being overheard	High	NCT 2003
Freedom to do what feels right during labour and delivery	High	Boulton, Chapple & Saunders 2003

as aromatherapy, music and visually interesting outlooks including windows with views, flowers, plants, tropical fish tanks and water features were suggested as ways of enhancing birth environments (NCT 2003).

While the NCT (2003) study focused on how the environment affects women's birth experience, Lock and Gibb (2003) sought to discover how the location for postnatal care (home or hospital) impacted women's experience. The findings of this Australian study emphasize that 'place' as a construct involves power issues since wherever events such as birth or the postnatal experience are located, that is 'someone's territory'. When the 'territory' is a hospital, the experience is overlayed with the hospital's physical appearance and layout, plus unwritten rules and constraints. In the hospital, women were 'given a bed' and had to adapt to a 'harsh, confined physical world' which was 'horrible' with 'plastic up the walls'. One woman described in dismay her 'one window [that had]...Venetian blinds and I couldn't see out the window' (Lock and Gibb 2003, p. 135). Women said that when they were at home, acknowledged as a place of comfort, they could be 'themselves'. Hospital as a place of birth was identified as a place of physical safety, but not emotional safety as the women in this study were at 'risk of becoming enculturated into dependence' (Lock and Gibb 2003, p. 136). Mothers felt they had to leave hospital as quickly as possible after the birth lest they became 'sicker'.

Interestingly, while the NCT study demonstrated that women want control and seek independence, safety was not mentioned as an important element in the physical environment. Physical safety may have been something the women in the NCT study took for granted and instead were focusing on emotional safety. Risk and safety are concepts that are influenced by the environment that people find themselves in. Mead and Kornbrodt (2004) found that midwive's perception of 'risk' was at odds with reality as it was increased when they worked in environments in which high levels of intervention were practised. It would appear that rather than being stress reducing, the 'high tech' environment appeared to raise levels of anxiety. In this way 'high tech' environments can increase the perception of risk and therefore intervention. In 'low tech' environments midwives' perception of risk is more realistic resulting in low intervention. Perhaps this result provides an insight into how women may respond to a 'high tech' or 'low tech' physical environment for birth.

There is a steadily growing body of knowledge that strongly suggests the way healthcare facilities look, feel and function has an impact on stress as humans are hard wired to be responsive and sensitive to everything in their environment (Shur Bilchik 2002). A calming environment has been established as one that incorporates a focus on nature. A plausible explanation of why a focus on nature is calming and stress reducing can be found by considering the implications of the biophilia hypothesis proposed by a Harvard entomologist, Edward Wilson in 1984 (Gullone 2000).

THE BIOPHILIA HYPOTHESIS

This hypothesis proposes that as a consequence of evolution human beings have developed an innate tendency to affiliate with nature. Humans focus on life and environmental stimuli that are life giving and consequently are also aesthetically pleasing. Cross-cultural evolutionary research has revealed our psychological wellbeing is increased when we are exposed to natural features in the environment. We have preferences for particular features such as water (essential for all life); savannah (rather than dense forest since the savannah is where there is usually a plentiful food supply and the savannah is more conducive to detecting predators); trees with either low trunks (could be climbed in times of danger) or trees with high canopies (did not block the view and enemies could not hide behind them); looking down on the grasslands from a higher place (again protective against predators so is life giving, but also provides a view of animals below who provide a food source); and we have an innate aversion to certain stimuli such as spiders, snakes, heights, dogs, sharks – and enclosed spaces (possibly because we cannot escape if we needed to) (Gullone 2000). These preferences and aversions have evolved during our long history as subsistence, hunters, gatherers and farmers and are a 'deep defining part of human evolutionary experience that has become genetically encoded to enhance survival and reproductive fitness' (Gullone 2000, p. 294). It is therefore reasonable to propose that the natural environment has also shaped our cognitive and emotional brain. Much of the tendency to biophilia is still present within us and appears in all cultures in symbolic ways. It is suggested that oral folklore and mythology have evolved to facilitate these adaptive processes.

What does this have to do with the birth environment you may ask? We suggest two things. The first is that researchers in this field have established that we have not yet developed an inbuilt aversion to man-made dangerous objects (such as firearms or frayed electric cords for example). This suggests that our adaptive responses have not yet caught up with the unprecedented human manufactured change that has occurred in Western societies over the last 200 years. We now find ourselves in man made environments that our ancestors could not have imagined. We need to consider that humans do not have an unlimited capacity to adapt to environments that are far removed from that in which we evolved. Arguably evolutionary change takes much longer than 200 years. This raises a number of questions about the impact of man-made birth environments, which house most Western women during childbirth. We need to compare these birthplaces with what, in evolutionary terms, might be seen as the ideal. The second is the importance of an engagement with nature during pregnancy, labour and birth in order to enhance maternal and infant physical and psychological wellbeing and to reduce stress. Maternal and infant biology has not changed as quickly or as much as the environments in which our biology unfolds. By recognizing these differences we can act to ameliorate some of the differences between ancient and recent environments to improve maternal and infant wellbeing (Trevathan and McKenna 1994).

An examination of birth environments across non-western cultures and where technology and medicalized birth is less evident, reveals many common features. Birth usually always takes place in the presence of another familiar person. Women rarely choose to birth alone or with strangers. It is rare to find women who give birth in unfamiliar surroundings preferring instead their own home, or that of a close relative or 'in-law'. Occasionally women birth in a specially built structure such as the menstrual hut found in some societies and rarely, but occasionally, women birth out in the open (Engelmann 1884). In all cultures, a wide range of activities are associated with birth with the goal of reassuring the mother and endeavouring to ease the process with massages, herbal teas, rituals and activities including music and chanting. The woman is free to move about at her will during the labour and for the actual birth may squat, kneel or sit in a special bed or chair. Another person, who sits or stands behind her, always supports the woman. All cultures have an experienced birth attendant, usually a woman, and often attendance at birth is restricted to women. However, even cross cultural descriptions of the place of birth provide only cursory details of the components of the space.

BIRTH CENTRES

One response to the stressful, anxiety-inducing man-made birth environment has been the development of the family birth centre and much has been written about birth centres over the years (Hofmeyr et al 1991; Fannin 2003; Kirkham 2003; Walsh 2007). However, almost all studies have focused on identifying clinical, psychosocial and economic outcomes of birth centres, with few revealing any descriptions of their physical design and structure. One recent, comprehensive review found no standard definition of a birth centre existed, although the authors did differentiate between freestanding units and those alongside hospital obstetric units (Stewart et al 2004). While the review incorporated 34 studies revealing that birth centre care offers the possibility of accessible, appropriate, personal maternity care for women and their families it did not provide any description of the physical attributes of birth centres themselves.

In evaluating a new service at a birth centre in Edgware in the UK, researchers asked women who used the service to rate the features that were most important to them (Boulton et al 2003). The top three features identified were 'the relaxed and homely atmosphere; having their own room and the freedom to do what feels right during labour and delivery'. The elements of what constituted a 'relaxed and homely atmosphere' were not specified in the article. In discussing the attributes which make a birth centre attractive to birthing women, Walsh (2007) also fails to examine the physical attributes of the space. He suggests that in seeking to make the centre homelike and an 'oasis of calm' and a 'nurturing environment', birthing centres may be operating out of a 'vicarious nesting instinct'. In this way, it can feel right for women to have their babies at the centre and therefore trigger the woman's innate, intuitive nesting instinct. Walsh quotes one woman who said 'the birth space is somewhere you could relax' and another said 'I could picture myself there'.

One of the newest birth centres in Australia is the Belmont Birthing Service in New South Wales. One of us (CH) is currently the manager of the service so we have an in-depth knowledge of its design and function. The Birth Centre came about because the obstetric service in the area closed due to a lack of available paediatricians and anaesthetists. However, local women demanded to be provided with a local maternity service. Despite strong opposition from some medical practitioners, the Area Health Service approved the establishment of a midwifery-managed, freestanding unit, which opened in July 2005. Using principles derived from Feng Shui, the midwives have created a place of beauty with a focus on nature. The feature walls are painted red, or green or purple in line with the chakras (see Table 7.1). There are numerous pieces of art (paintings and sculptures) containing birth and feminine archetypes throughout the building. Large oval baths are provided in the birth rooms. Plants, music, aromatherapy, open space, a water feature, and photographic displays of mothers, fathers and babies are some of the elements of the physical environment. The kitchen is a hub for many conversations; open to both midwives and parents with mealtimes shared around the table. A playroom for siblings, supplied with beautiful toys provided by the community of women, is located within the centre. The entry is lined with greenery. Women and their partners often comment how relaxed,

friendly and calming the environment feels. The vision of the service is 'enriching lives through positive birth experiences' and the midwives are committed to supporting women and their families through their transformative journeys. On entry to the midwifery service, the women and midwives negotiate an ethical agreement in line with that described in Chapter 3 of this book.

While the outcomes of the service (maternal and infant mortality and morbidity; maternal satisfaction; midwifery satisfaction; costs) are being evaluated, it is not possible to easily determine what effect the physical environment has separate to the model of midwifery care since both act synergistically. What is apparent is that the midwives in this setting are highly skilled, ontologically aware practitioners incorporating all aspects of mindbodyspirit and technological competencies into the birth territory. The Birth Centre midwives are what the eminent nursing scholar, Jean Watson (1999), would refer to as ontological architects. This is an important concept to consider.

MIDWIVES AS ONTOLOGICAL ARCHITECTS

Ontology refers to the meaning of 'being' and what it means to be human. Watson calls for an ontological shift in the caring sciences from a consciousness about 'being' which '...moves from "being human" implying separate, independent individuals, disconnected from self-other-environment-nature-universe, to reconsidering "being human" in relation with and seeking harmony with all else in the universe' (Watson 1999, p. 289). A midwife working as an ontological architect is aware that we (and the women for whom we care) breathe in our surroundings with all our senses moment to moment; that our conscious and unconscious perception of the environment has a powerful impact on our mindbodyspirit and that we need to pay conscious attention to creating spirit nourishing and healing spaces for birth to proceed optimally. This does not mean a rejection of medical science in favour of the arts in caring/healing. On the contrary, this will require us to develop professional ontological competencies which will prepare midwives with skills in both the technological aspects of practice (when needed) as well as the vision and knowledge to create and guard a sacred space in which women will feel enabled to give birth.

CONCLUSION

For centuries modern society has believed that using logic and rational scientific practices can solve all the problems of human life. This belief has become the foundation for all fields of intellectual inquiry in the sciences, medicine, engineering, architecture and other endeavours. As a result, a style of architecture has developed that is characterized by anonymous apartment blocks and rows of identical, isolated, bland, suburban houses. Recently modern architecture has been called to task for creating buildings that have been vilified as nothing but 'warehouses for bodies' that increase our disconnection from and relationship with nature and each other (Watson 1999). The sight of one community so horrified American song writer Malvina Reynolds that she was moved to write the song 'Little Boxes' that lampoons the development of suburbia with its square, straight lines and sharp angled boxy structures made of 'ticky tacky', that are spiritually empty (Reynolds 1962).

These structures stand in stark contrast to pre-modern architecture with its more organic shapes and materials and to which societies are now returning. We have discovered that the relentless pursuit of rationality and logic has not only failed to solve many of the problems of human life but may in fact be responsible for their very creation. Modern architecture made up of rectangular forms and straight lines (which are found nowhere in the natural world or the living human body) has been described as 'death to the soul' and environments that are '...faceless, harsh and sterile can actually make us feel unwell, exhausted and disconnected with our energy source and ourselves' (Watson 1999, p. 243). Postmodern architecture is now reintroducing '...elements of beauty, local colour, decoration, historical references and even playfulness and fantasy... full of cultural meaning' into the exterior and interior of public and private spaces (Watson 1999, p. 245). In health care, this has inspired a new generation of architectural thinking that seeks to build spirit nourishing, spatial and sensory buildings that

exemplify caring/healing and employing a range of healing art modalities.

Since Roger Ulrich's discovery in 1984 that postsurgical patients whose rooms offered an outdoor view recovered more quickly, researchers with an interest in caring/healing arts and architecture have begun to systematically explore the impact of the environment on health and healing, at least for short-term outcomes (Marcelis et al 1998; Shur Bilchik 2002). For example, several studies in the area of music and healing have established that the growth of cells within tumours are significantly decreased when exposed to primordial sounds (such as a heart beat or intake of breath or the sound of running water) and increased when exposed to rock music (Sharma et al 1996). Singing lullabies to premature infants in an intensive care unit has been found to decrease the length of hospital stay by 3 days when compared to infants in a control group who were not exposed to the singing (Coleman et al 1994). Movement such as dance or Tai Chi has been found to improve the wellbeing of elderly people (Scott et al 2001). A World Symposium on Culture, Health and the Arts held at Manchester Metropolitan University in 1999 examined the therapeutic benefits of landscapes and gardens and the effects of art on a range of health outcomes (Friedrich 1999). However, we have been unable to locate any studies that have attempted to explore the impact of mindbodyspirit birth architecture on birth outcomes.

It is no longer possible to simply dismiss the bricks and mortar of the birth space as irrelevant to the processes and outcomes of birth. Studies that attempt to evaluate the effectiveness of birth centres compared with standard birth spaces will need to 'operationalize' the concept 'birth space' in each location in order to make robust comparisons and draw meaningful conclusions about differences in outcomes. Many past studies have failed to consider the impact of the physical environment for birth and have merely focussed on the model of care and/or women's perceptions of personal control, safety and satisfaction in each location. Comparisons of home and hospital birth are similarly flawed since it is now clear that there are important elements in each space that will impact mindbodyspirit physiology that have not been assessed.

Investigating the impact of mindbodyspirit design principles provides a new and exciting research agenda for the future since many maternity units are undergoing renewal and rebuilding projects which can utilize these concepts. Evaluating the impact of the new designs must be an integral part of the process. Whether simply adding mindbodyspirit considerations to existing birth spaces will make a difference to outcomes can similarly be evaluated. National guidelines for the design and construction of hospitals and health care facilities will need to be radically reviewed and redeveloped to encompass mindbodyspirit principles rather than focusing on the limited repertoire of setting spatial and safety dimensions for conducting procedures to rectify pathology. An integrated mindbodyspirit design together with health-care providers who understand and act ontologically will provide optimal birth spaces for women and babies.

References

Boulton M, Chapple J, Saunders D 2003 Evaluating a new service: Clinical outcomes and women's assessments of the Edgware Birth Centre. In: M Kirkham (Ed). Birth centres: A social model for maternity care. Books for Midwives. Elsevier Science, London.

Canetti E 1983 La provincia dell'uomo. Adelphi, Milan.

Coleman JH, Pratt RR, Stoddard RA, Gerstmann D, Abel HH 1994 The effects of the male and female singing voices on selected physiological and behavioural measures of premature infants in the intensive care unit. International Journal of Alternative Medicine 5(2): 4–11.

Coyle K, Hauck Y, Percival P, Kristjanson L 2001 Ongoing relationships with a personal focus: mother's perceptions of birth centre versus hospital care. Midwifery 17: 171–181.

Foureur M 2003 A survey of women's expectations and experience of the environment for birth, Wellington New Zealand. Unpublished Health Service Survey.

Engelmann GJ 1884 Labor among primitive peoples. JH Chambers & Co, St Louis, accessed from http://etext.lib.virginia.edu/modeng/modengE.browse.html

Emslie MJ, Campbell MK, Walker KA, Robertson S, Campbell A 1999 Developing consumer-led maternity services: A survey of women's views in a local healthcare setting. Health Expectations 2: 195–207.

Fannin M 2003 Domesticating Birth in the hospital: family centred birth and the emergence of homelike birthing rooms. Antipode 35(5): 1039–1042 doi:10.1111/j.1467-8330.2003.00376.x.

Fenwick J, Hauck Y, Downie J, Butt J 2004 The childbirth expectations of a self-selected cohort of Western Australian women. Midwifery 21(1): 23–35.

Franck K, Lepori B 2007 Architecture inside out. Wiley Edition, London.

Fraser D, Watts K, Munir F 2003 Under the spotlight: Grantham's midwife-managed unit. In: M Kirkham (Ed). Birth centres: A social model for maternity care. Books for Midwives. Elsevier Science, London.

Freidrich MJ 1999 The arts of healing. Journal of American Medical Association 181(19): 1779–1781.

Gullone E 2000 The biophilia hypothesis and life in the 21st century: Increasing mental health or increasing pathology? Journal of Happiness Studies 1: 293–321.

Handler A, Raube K, Kelley MA, Giachello A 1996 Women's satisfaction with prenatal care settings: A focus group study. Birth 23(1): 31–37.

Hodnett ED, Downe S, Edwards N, Walsh D 2005 Home-like versus conventional institutional settings for birth. The Cochrane Database of Systematic Reviews 1. Art No.:CD000012.pub2.DOI:10.1002/14651858. CD000012.pub2

Hofmeyr G, Nikodem V, Wolman W, Chalmers E, Kramer T 1991 Companionship to modify the clinical Birth Environment: Effects on progress and perceptions of labour, and breastfeeding. British Journal of Obstetrics and Gynaecology 98(8): 756–64.

Kaufman K 2000 Commentary: Have we yet learned about the effects of continuity of midwifery care? Birth 27(3): 174–176.

Kirkham M 2003 Birth centres: A social model for maternity care. Books for Midwives. Elsevier Science, London.

Lepori B 1992 La nascita e i suoi luoghi. Red edizioni, Como.

Lepori B 1994 Freedom of movement in birth places. Children's environments 11(2): 81–87.

Lock LR, Gibb HJ 2003 The power of place. Midwifery 19:132–139.

Marcelis M, Navarro-Mateu F, Murray R, Selten J, Van Os J 1998 Urbanization and psychosis: A study of 1942–1978 birth cohorts in The Netherlands. Psychological Medicine 28: 871–879.

Mead MMP, Kornbrot D 2004 The influence of maternity units' intrapartum intervention rates and midwives' risk perception for women suitable for midwifery led care. Midwifery 20: 61–71.

National Childbirth Trust Annual Conference 2003 Building for a Better Birth. London.

Rennie AM, Hundley V, Gurney E, Graham W 1998 Women's priorities for care before and after delivery. British Journal of Midwifery 6(7): 434–438.

Reynolds M 1962 Little Boxes. Schroder Music Company, Berkeley.

Scott AH, Butin DN, Tewfik D et al 2001 Occupational therapy as a means to wellness with the elderly. Physical and Occupational Therapy in Geriatrics 18(4): 3–22.

Sharma HM, Kauffman EM, Stephens RE 1996 Effect of different sounds on growth of human cancer cells lines in vitro. Alternative Therapies in Clinical Practice 3(4): 25–32.

Shur Blichuk G 2002 A better place to heal. Health Forum Journal July/August: 10–15.

Singh D, Newburn M 2006 Feathering the nest: What women want from the birth environment. RCM Midwives Journal 9(7): 266–269.

Stewart M, McCandlish R, Henderson J, Brockhurst P 2004 Report of a structured review of birth centre outcomes. National Perinatal Epidemiology Unit, Oxford.

Trevathan WR, McKenna J 1994 Evolutionary environments of human birth and infancy: Insights to apply to contemporary life. Children's Environments 11(2): 13–36.

Walsh D, Downe S 2004 Outcomes of free-standing, midwife-led birth centers: A structured review. Birth 31(3): 222.

Walsh D 2005 Subverting the assembly-line: Childbirth in a free-standing birth centre. Social Science and Medicine 62: 1330–1340.

Walsh D 2007 Improving maternity services: Small is beautiful – lessons from a birth centre. Radcliffe Publishing, Seattle.

Watson J 1999 Postmodern nursing and beyond. Churchill Livingstone, Edinburgh.

Wiegers TA, Keirse MJN, van der Zee J, Berg GAH 1996 Outcome of planned home and hospital births in low risk pregnancies: Prospective study in midwifery practices in the Netherlands. British Medical Journal 313: 1309–1313.

Section **3**

Midwives, obstetricians and the maternity services

SECTION CONTENTS

Chapter **8**

Being a midwife to midwifery: Transforming midwifery services

Lesley Page

INTRODUCTION

Imagine two different maternity services. Imagine one service that is very good, and one that is dysfunctional. In the first women are cared for in both community and hospital by a midwife they will get to know and trust, and who will provide most of their care. The woman's named midwife works with one or two other midwives. Midwives take full responsibility for care unless there is a medical problem. If they need to refer to a doctor the relationship is respectful. These midwifery practices are embedded into group practices providing support for each other. Although they may practice differently to other core midwives who are working in wards and departments not providing continuity there is integration in that each respects and understands the role of the other. There are clear systems of referral between midwives and with medical staff. There is a strong interface between hospital and community.

All staff in this 'good' service will get the opportunity to keep their skills and knowledge up to date, and discussion and questioning in meetings and the clinical area keeps the ethos dynamic. The values and aims of the service are clear and known by all staff. There are resources for teaching and learning, systems for support, and staff feel comfortable asking for help if they are unsure or lack confidence. Some midwives provide care for women through the whole process following women through the system, and some are on the core staff, providing support to their colleagues. The physical environment provides bright clean rooms in which women can move, be comfortable, use water for labour and birth, and have privacy.

In the second service, that I will describe as dysfunctional, women are seen by a number of different midwives and doctors. Care is fragmented. There are not enough midwives and roles between midwives, doctors and perhaps nurses are confused. There is little time for education and development. Values, aims and philosophy are unclear. There may be too many meetings but there is little real talk; in meetings there is little real exchange of opinions. There may be a divide between management and staff. When staff join the service there is little orientation as there is a shortage of staff. Midwives start work before they know the ropes, and there are few colleagues who can be called on to help. The atmosphere is full of anxiety. While on the surface people seem to get on there may be bullying and fearful relationships. In the hospital rooms are crowded and it is difficult for women to get comfortable. The hospital may well be dirty. It may be difficult for women to get a home birth, or to make decisions about their care.

I hope you can see these services through the eyes of a woman who is expecting a baby, and through the eyes of a midwife, perhaps just starting to work there. Each of them, both the woman and the midwife, has expectations and anxieties. For both the quality of the service, that is the culture and ethos of the organization, the staff relationships, the availability of resources, the physical environment, standards of practice, ethics of care and leadership and management, and support for learning and development, will make a huge difference. For women their ability to develop a trusting relationship with individual midwives, to feel that their care is of the utmost importance, that midwives are skilled and knowledgeable, will make a profound difference to their experience of care and the outcomes of birth. For the midwife, the service she works in may enable her to practice fully as a midwife, or will make this very difficult. The midwife is guardian of the woman's care and experience of birth, as well as the outcomes. The maternity service is the foundation for the care the midwife provides.

The leaders of midwifery in that service are in their turn the guardians of the potential for midwives to do their best for the women and families in their care, they are midwives to other midwives, working with them rather than over them, creating a situation in which they may practice and develop to the full. The maternity services, that are shaped to a great extent, but not entirely, by the leaders within them, should help midwives provide care that is not only effective, but also sensitive to the needs of women and their families. They should help create services in which the needs of individual women, and communities served, are uppermost, what is often called woman-centred care. This sensitivity is best achieved by trusting relationships in which women and their midwives may get to know each other over time, relationships in which continuity is a characteristic. In turn midwives need to work in functional, supportive and trusting relationships with each other and with other staff. In addition to this the service needs to run smoothly and efficiently for midwives (and all staff) to be able to give of their best.

In this chapter I will describe some of the problems that have arisen in modern maternity services that have prevented midwives from being effective and sensitive, and why they have arisen. I will describe the need for the creation of change, and will describe the characteristics of what is called The New Midwifery (Page and McCandlish 2006) and the importance of effective sensitive midwifery to what is a critical period in human life.

The basic argument of this chapter is that the organizations in which midwives practice should enable the creation of the new midwifery, but that often the maternity services in which the majority of midwives practice make it very difficult to practice effectively. Drawing on theory, evidence and experience the chapter will propose ways of making the maternity services better for midwives, in order that they may support women and their families, and local childbearing communities more appropriately.

THE SIGNIFICANCE OF BIRTH

Pregnancy, birth, and the early weeks of human life are a time of profound significance. This is a critical point in the life of the newborn, the parents and the family. Sensitive effective care given at this time will affect not only physical health but also sense of self and competence as a mother and father, feelings of love for the baby, and memories of the experience of care. Positive care will make a huge difference to the outcome. Negative care is perhaps more powerful and may increase a lifetime of problems in relationships, or physical problems, and may make the difference between life and death. Both good and bad care will be remembered. The care of the individual family will have reverberations into communities and society. Good care around the time of birth is important to all of life (McCourt, Hirst and Page 2000; Page 2004; Redshaw 2006).

THE NEW MIDWIFERY – WORKING WITH WOMEN

To be a midwife means being able to work with a woman, in the sense of working alongside her, to ensure that the care we offer meets her individual needs and those of her family in the early weeks of family life. Being a midwife 'with the woman' implies a relationship of knowing each other, of mutual trust, of working in the best interests of the woman and her family and ensuring that their care is uppermost in midwifery work.

The essence of midwifery is to assist women around the time of childbirth, in ways that recognize that the physical, emotional and spiritual aspects of pregnancy and birth are equally important. Midwifery care is likely to have profound and long-term consequences not only on physical outcomes, but also on personal and family integrity, and the relationship between mother and her partner and the baby. Of course a midwife must provide competent and safe physical care – but without sacrificing respect for the emotional and spiritual dimensions which give meaning to the whole individual and personal experience of pregnancy and birth.

In her everyday and intimate connection with birth, a midwife is the guardian of one of life's most important events, for each individual and for society as a whole. Being a midwife, being 'with woman' is a privileged role; one which a wealth of art and science, knowledge and expertise, humanity and spirit surround and which combine to bring a unique and irreplaceable approach to care.

The new midwifery consists of five essential characteristics:

- Working in a positive relationship with women.
- Being aware of the significance of pregnancy and birth and the early weeks of life as the start of human life and the new family.
- Avoiding harm by using the best information or evidence in practice.
- Having adequate skills to deliver effective care and support.
- Promoting health and wellbeing.

(Page and McCandlish 2006, with permission.)

In order to practice the new midwifery midwives need the appropriate support and context for care. As modern maternity services have developed in industrialized societies the traditional meaning of midwifery has been lost. The new midwifery is a concept that integrates the traditional meaning of midwifery with the kind of midwifery that is related to modern day maternity services.

The effect of the culture and organization of maternity services

Why should the difficulty of practising to their full potential have arisen for midwives in modern industrialized societies? How have midwives become uprooted from the essential concept of the word to be 'with woman'? How might midwives start to work with women again rather than with institution? It is important to understand the basis of the problem if we are to resolve it.

The word midwife is Anglo-Saxon meaning 'with the woman'. Until the middle of the 20th century in the UK and many other parts of the world midwives remained a part of the communities in which women lived. Although history marks the beginning of the erosion of the midwife's role with the development of obstetric forceps by Chamberlain (the professionalization of midwifery in 1902 in the UK was seen by some as a means of controlling the profession by doctors), it was perhaps the movement of birth from the home to the hospital that made the most fundamental changes to midwifery.

While birth was community and home-based, midwives were in touch with the everyday lives of women, and were able to work in some kind of continuous relationship with them. Stevens (2003) describes the midwife as 'a known and trusted community figure'. With the movement of birth to the hospital, the majority of midwives started to practice in the hospital setting. Allocated to wards and departments rather than being responsible for the care of a community of women, care became fragmented. As the number of medical interventions in birth increased, so the possibility of midwifery autonomy decreased. By the late 1970s most midwives were 'independent practitioners in their own right' in name only, although a small number of independent and community midwives continued to work in relationship with individual women, utilizing all of their skills and knowledge. The majority of midwives experienced little autonomy, and the role of midwifery had become confused with the role of nursing. Often not only professional autonomy but also any sense of a professional role was lost. For example many midwives in the UK acted solely as receptionists in clinics for much of their time.

The move to universal hospitalization in the industrialized Western world, to almost routine induction of labour in the 1970s, to systems where women were routinely shaved and given enemas in labour, continued into the 1970s. During the 1970s and 1980s the real problems being experienced in the maternity services were becoming apparent. Despite the improving perinatal mortality rates, there was a seemingly paradoxical sense of discontent among women and the frustration of midwives with the increasing limitation of their roles was becoming obvious (Robinson 1989). Not only was there an increasing rate of medical intervention, inductions, epidurals and operative births, but the organization of midwifery, on an acute nursing model, was not appropriate to midwifery. Midwives could not follow women through the process of care; neither could they maintain all of their skills. In most services in the UK a process of rotation was developed in order to ensure that midwives could maintain their skills in all areas. This however, meant that midwives moved from one area to another, meaning that they had no 'home' and there were no stable teams of midwives. This made it difficult for team work or team development because there was no stability.

There are a number of theories or theoretical perspectives that may be used to explain the sense of frustration of midwives and the dysfunctional organizations and culture of care that exist to this day (Hunt and Symonds 1995; Barclay and Jones 1996; House of Commons (HOC) 2003a,b,c;). There are of course powerful political and social factors that affect our approach to birth and to midwifery. These theories include the simple explanation of the way the structure of care, that is fragmented care, has separated women from their midwives, to theories about the behaviour of oppressed groups (Kirkham and Stapleton (2001, 2004)), to psychoanalytical theories about the maladaptive containment of anxiety (Menzies 1988), to theories about a technocratic culture of care (Davis-Floyd 2001).

The work of Menzies holds some resonance for me (Menzies 1988). Menzie's work, that arose from nursing in the 1960s, seems to help to explain the frustration and alienation experienced by many midwives, and the difficulty of retaining and attracting midwives to practice. Working from a psychoanalytical perspective, Menzies proposed that in their contact with illness, death and dying, pain and other extremely distressing situations, nurses had to confront their most primal anxieties. In order to contain their anxieties nurses chose a maladaptive response. Rather than confronting their fears and anxieties and building structures that allowed them to support those they cared for, they separated themselves by developing hierarchical and task oriented care, thus avoiding the need to confront their extreme anxieties.

With the move from home to hospital, midwives took on nursing structures and the hierarchical task oriented approach of nursing at that time. Although this theory may explain destructive effects to nursing the effect on midwifery may have been more pronounced. Midwives, who were to leave behind a tradition of being part of the communities of women they cared for with the hospitalization of birth, moved into structures of care where separation of women and their midwives was institutionalized in the hospital. As with nurses this maladaptive way of containing anxiety by socially constructed defence mechanisms may have led to unresolved tensions and increased frustration for midwives as well as women, and an inevitable alienation. A more effective way of resolving the anxieties engendered by facing intense and often difficult situations is to work to reduce the anxiety by recognizing it and supporting those being cared for, while recognizing the complexity of problems that are inherent, and require complex problem solving in turn.

The work of Kirkham and Stapleton (2004) has been invaluable in helping to understand the prevailing culture of midwifery in the National Health Service in the UK that may be similar to the culture of other health services (Brodie 1996). Citing (KirKham and Stapleton, 2001, p.157) the work of Heagarty, Kirkham, Witz, Davies, Bologh, Freire and Roberts they described how: 'In less than a century English midwives became regulated, professionalized and medically controlled. The values reflected in the organization of midwives were those of an organizational vision culturally coded as masculine. The domestic, caring female values became increasingly invisible, although remained essential, in the support of individual childbearing women. Adjusting to profound changes, midwives manifest the classic responses of an oppressed group, internalizing the powerful values of medicine and exercising 'horizontal violence' towards colleagues seen as deviant.' It is easy to see then, that the support of women in having choice and control of their own care, pregnancy and birth by midwives, may be limited in a profession that sees itself as powerless, and will control other members of the profession who are seeking change, and endeavouring to empower childbearing women.

GUARDING THE MIDWIFE

The nature of the maternity services in which midwives practice will vary between different countries. In large part the nature is determined by the characteristics of the health service, but also by other cultural norms (Page 2003a). While in a number of countries midwives may practice outside of, but linked to, the hospital system, the large number of midwives in the industrialized world will practise within hospitals, or within services that bridge hospital and community. The maternity service as a whole should provide for care in the woman's own community, including home birth, one of the safest places to give birth where the pregnancy is low risk and there is the back-up of a hospital system and emergency services (Page 2006b). We are becoming more aware of the negative effects of poverty; it is one of the biggest risk factors for childbearing women and their babies. Thus public health approaches, and being integrated into local communities, becomes even more important (Chapple 2006; Dunkley-Bent 2006).

The autonomy of midwives is likely to be greater where they are not employed by the maternity service, but work in a strong interface with it (Page 2003a). In the Netherlands, parts of Canada, and New Zealand, midwives may practice independently but also as part of the health service, while having admitting privileges to hospital, and the right of referral to obstetricians. Where midwives are employed directly by the maternity service there have been a number of developments in many parts of the world to enable midwives to follow women through the whole process of care, working in community and hospital. These continuity of care schemes or caseload models are focused on enabling midwives to work in relationship with women, and to practice their skills fully (Page 2003b, 2004).

Wherever midwives work there are universal principles that will support the midwife to do her best, as Curtis Ball and Kirkham put it 'to be the midwife she wants to be' (2006). Generally, the interests of childbearing women and their midwives are mutual; what serves one group will serve the other. Midwives need to be supported in order to support women. The work of redeveloping midwifery has started in many parts of the world. In general this work may consist of three different but interrelated elements:

- Restructuring or redesigning services to enable continuity of carer.
- Developing an appropriate organizational culture with clear values and philosophy (transformational change).
- Ensuring an efficient well-run service.

The remainder of this chapter will discuss change that falls in these three areas.

ENABLING GOOD MIDWIFERY: HELPING MIDWIVES TO WORK WITH WOMAN

The new midwifery is founded on the 'with woman' relationship. This implies a relationship in which each learns to trust the other, there is reciprocity in the relationship, and the midwife works in the best interests of the woman. Pairman asserts that midwifery *is* the relationship (Pairman 2006). Others have found that a meaningful relationship with women is one of the factors that provides satisfaction for midwives, and makes them want to stay in the profession (Sandall 1997, 2003; Kirkham and Stapleton (2001, 2004); Deery and Kirkham 2006). In addition, Sandall describes the need for occupational autonomy, social support and developing meaningful relationships with women (1997, p. 106).

Continuity – an essential aspect of relationship

Work to reinstate the relationship between women and their midwives, the development of what was called at that time simply 'continuity of care' or team midwifery began in the UK in late 1960s and 1970s (Seccombe and Stock 1995). By continuity of care I mean the provision of a system of care where women are cared for by a named midwife who provides most of her care, with the named midwife being supported by one or a small group of other midwives to allow time off. The central aim of continuity of care is to enable the development of a relationship of trust that is reciprocal between women and their midwives.

In contrast, team midwifery indicates that the emphasis is on providing care for groups of women by a team of midwives. There are other definitions and the lack of agreed definition has created many problems. Interest in the reorganization of care grew with growing dissatisfaction with care (Seccombe and Stock 1995). About this time the Association of Radical Midwives published The Vision (Association of Radical Midwives 1986). The Grace Project (Weatherston 1985) and the Know your Midwife project (Flint and Poulengeris 1987) had developed on different sides of the Atlantic. The scholarly work of analysing the nature of the relationship to be developed in these new patterns of practice had only just started at the time. There was an assumption that was held by many of us developing 'continuity of care' schemes, that the continuing and continuous midwifery relationship was fundamental and would lead to increased satisfaction for women, and would decrease the intervention rates associated with birth. The concept of continuity of care was the catch-all phrase for developments in midwifery that were seen by many as the essential and necessary solution to many of the problems of midwifery, and crucial to the building of more humane, individualized maternity services. But the assumptions of many of us who undertook the work of developing continuity of care were that others would understand what this brief managerial phrase meant implicitly to us. To this day misunderstanding of what continuity of care means creates problems, in lack of clarity about what is to be achieved when establishing new systems of midwifery practice, and in the evaluation and interpretation of research findings. However, we are now getting a little closer to some conceptual clarity and an understanding of how and why continuity of care is important to women and to midwives (Page 2004).

It is important then to go no further until the concept of continuity of care is defined, and the purpose made clear. Because the purpose of this relationship is, as I see it, to support the power of the childbearing woman, I will start with the words of women themselves, then move to a more academic definition and explanatory theories of why continuity of care works.

What continuity means to women
Maureen Freeley, a well-known journalist in the UK, wrote of her early experience of team midwifery, established at the John Radcliffe in Oxford in the late 1980s. She wrote also of other experiences of fragmented care in the standard service that team midwifery had replaced. She saw the continuity provided by team midwifery as taking the long view, of increasing the safety of care. Freeley (1995) wrote, 'after the placenta had been delivered, I felt strong enough to have a shower, and then it was up to the ward where I watched the other new mothers being subjected to the indifferent care of midwives on the shift, while I continued to get what looked

like special treatment from the team midwives. In fact, if you added up the minutes of care we received, I probably took less time to care for, simply because my midwives knew who I was and what I had been through and so could use the shorthand of a working friendship...If the midwife had been a total stranger I might have been too embarrassed to ask her for help...but because trust was so well established I didn't think twice about it...why...because the care I received from them was care with a face and a memory and an ever-open ear. It made me feel like an active participant-and not as I had been on many other occasions, a vessel at the mercy of experts. It was not just woman-centred. It was man-centred. It was home and family-centred even when we were in the hospital' (pp. 6–7).

Freeley (1995) articulated and illustrated the principles clearly. The words of women that follow, recorded by a researcher, about their experience of one-to-one midwifery care, placed intentionally in a very deprived area, were just as, if not more, compelling, showing as they do a lack of familiarity with English.

> 'I knew exactly what was going to happen, when and how, that was one bit of it. Another thing is you knew the person there, and she was there only herself, no-one else'.

Another woman said:

> 'Well I could talk to her about anything and say to her everything, that's how much confidence I had in her' (McCourt, Hirst and Page 2000, p. 282).

Women do not generally use the terminology of continuity of care that is so familiar to midwives, but talked instead of the value of knowing their carers and why it was so important to them (McCourt, Hirst and Page 2000, p. 282). We see in the comments made by women the concepts of friendship, of trust, of intimacy, of feeling in control and informed, of confidence in the midwife.

A recent paper 'Continuity of care: A multidisciplinary review' (Haggerty et al 2003) describes three types of continuity:

- Informational continuity – the use of information on past events and personal circumstances to make current care appropriate for each individual.

- Management continuity – a consistent and coherent approach to the management of a health condition that is responsive to a patient's changing needs.
- Relational continuity – an ongoing therapeutic relationship between a patient and one or more providers.

In discussing relational continuity within primary care the main view of continuity as 'the relationship between a single practitioner and a patient that extends beyond a specific episode of illness or disease...implies a sense of loyalty by the patient and clinical responsibility by the provider...it fosters improved communication, trust and a sustained sense of responsibility' (Haggerty et al 2003, pp. 1219–1221).

This value based sense of loyalty and responsibility mirrors the experience of many in midwifery practice. What differentiates continuity of care in midwifery is the context of care: that is the care of women around the time of birth that is not simply a health event or an illness but an event of fundamental importance to all, with important emotional, social and spiritual meanings (Page 1989, 2004).

Help with understanding and conceptualizing continuity, and thus with putting it into operation, is aided by the hierarchy developed by Saultz and adapted by McCourt, et al (2006).

Hierarchical definition of continuity of care

The level of continuity, and their descriptions, is adapted from (Saultz 2003):

1. **Informational level**
   An organized collection of medical and social information about each woman is readily available to any healthcare professional caring for her. A systematic process also allows accessing and communicating about this information among those involved in the care.
2. **Longitudinal level**
   In addition to informational continuity, each woman has a 'place' where she receives most care, which allows the care to occur in an accessible and familiar environment from an organized team of providers. This team

assumes responsibility for coordinating the quality of care, including preventive services.

3. **Interpersonal level**

   In addition to longitudinal continuity, an ongoing relationship exists between each woman and a midwife. The woman knows the midwife by name and has come to trust the midwife on a personal basis. The woman uses this personal midwife for basic midwifery care and depends on the midwife to assume personal responsibility for her overall care. When the personal midwife is not available, coverage arrangement assures that longitudinal continuity occurs.

By arranging these concepts as a hierarchy, it is implied that at least some informational continuity is required for longitudinal continuity to be present and that longitudinal continuity is required for interpersonal continuity to exist in a midwife-woman relationship McCourt et al (2006) p. 143–144.

Continuity and associated outcomes

Outcomes of studies show an association between a decreased rate of interventions in pregnancy and birth and a high level of continuity of care (Page 2004). Davis-Floyd (2001) described the technocratic model that assumes a separation between mind and body. Interestingly where women have had a good relationship with a midwife they describe the confidence that this provides. Given that the reproductive system is under the control of the autonomic nervous system it seems logical to assume that this confidence affects mind and body. One of these skills that are central is the ability to provide a calm and reassuring presence.

However, we should not lose sight of the fact that this special relationship between the woman and her midwife is seen as an end in itself by many childbearing women, it is not purely functional (Page 2003a,b; 2004).

WHAT THE RELATIONSHIP MEANS TO MIDWIVES

Because the relationship is, as Stevens (2003) describes so clearly, reciprocal, it is worth looking briefly at what the relationship means to midwives at this point. Stevens describes the responses of midwives practising in the One-to-One Midwifery

Practice who felt like 'real midwives' for the first time. Emphasising the ideas of responsibility and trust, Stevens elaborates on the idea of knowing and what it means.

Once the words of women and midwives who have had experience of getting to know each other over time are heard, the word continuity becomes clearly inadequate to describe the complexity of what happens in this reciprocal process of midwife and woman working together in a relationship of trust and support for each other.

This complexity is also demonstrated in a chapter describing the relationship between women and midwives as one of partnership, and the development of trust and reciprocity, in the context of New Zealand, Pairman uses these words:

> '...She knew that I was scared, she knew how I was feeling. Because we discussed Lauren's birth in detail, and so she knew where I was coming from and I felt very comfortable with her...I trusted her totally' (2006, p. 88–89).

The relationship described by Pairman is one in which the midwife consciously helps the woman find her own power and support that may be translated to other areas of life, as these words show:

> 'It's a nice feeling to see a woman go from thinking that everyone else owns, or has a right to dictate, to deciding – and to see it spill over into other areas is really neat...and start questioning other areas and other things in her life...that's a major plus I think to work with a woman over a longer time' (2006, p. 90).

Empowering the midwife

In creating systems where midwives follow women through the whole system of care, being responsible for and having authority within the medical system to make clinical decisions together with the woman, a healthier adaptation to the reduction of anxiety is possible than the social defence mechanisms described by Menzies (1988). Of course the midwife must have the skills, knowledge, and aptitude to provide effective care. But rather than being alienated from those she cares for, she is in touch with women in a way that gives both the woman and the midwife together the agency to make appropriate decisions and act on them. So rather than a sense of free-floating anxiety, the midwife's concerns for the woman will not only be felt but may also be acted on. In addition, the evidence shows that there is intense satisfaction to be found not only for the woman but also for midwives practising in relationship with women.

However, it is particularly important that the organization provides support, not only for the woman, but also for the midwife, who will inevitably make some mistakes, and may well be involved in care where the baby may suffer long-term damage or die, or be involved in the care of families in extremely difficult circumstances and with horrendously difficult lives. (In my present service for example, in the centre of London, we care for women who are refugees from countries with extreme abuse of human rights, including torture, and women from war-torn countries who may have suffered multiple rape or even be pregnant as a result of rape, women who are extremely poor, and some who may be sex workers or substance abusers.)

Personal versus team caseload

A number of models have evolved over recent years that have ranged in the amount of continuity achieved. It is convenient here to divide them, somewhat simplistically, between those that have aimed to provide what has come to be called a 'team caseload'. Team midwifery is a team of midwives caring for a group of women and that is different from a 'personal caseload'. A personal caseload implies each woman having a named midwife who provides most of her care, with the named midwife being supported by one or a small number of partners. These differing systems may have different outcomes for women as well as midwives, and the differentiation in practice and research is crucial. The apparent attraction of team midwifery is easy to understand, because it appears to put less of an on call burden on individual midwives, and seems to be easier to arrange. However, it may not provide as many advantages to women, and may create problems for midwives (Sandall 1997). Innovations in care may also be divided into those that aim at increasing the autonomy of the midwife, by midwife-led care, rather than increasing continuity, and those that do both. One element of successful leadership and development is clarity about intention. This clarity in itself will be effective in achieving the desired aims.

Given that it may be the creation of reciprocal relationships in which women and midwives get to know and trust each other over time that is fundamental to a range of improved outcomes of care; it is not clear whether or not this is the intervention that has been evaluated in a number of the studies of continuity of care (Page 2004). Stevens (2003, p. 304) comments on the issue of minimal change and misleading evaluations. This is a crucial point. Many of the changes implemented have taken a 'tinkering at the edges' approach, presumably because it seems easier and less disruptive. However these schemes 'failed to embrace the fundamental change laid down by Winterton (House of Commons 1992) and The Expert Maternity Group (DOH 1993) [namely] that of replacing the medical model of childbirth with one that is woman-centred'. In Davis-Floyd's terms, this required replacing the technocratic model with a humanistic or even holistic model (2001).

Transforming practice – developing a positive culture of care

The restructure of services to enable continuity is not enough in itself. The restructure needs to be accompanied by change in the context of care, a transformation of the organization as a whole. Transformative change implies a change in the organization of care that goes beyond restructuring and superficial changes, that brings about clarification of purpose, clear values, and involvement of staff in the change (Page et al 1995; Page 2003a, 2004).

Woman-centred care is concerned with giving women and communities a place of power in the maternity services. By this I mean that women should be in control of what happens to them, and that services should be responsive to the needs of the local community, and include representatives of that community in planning and monitoring care. Making services accessible is particularly important to more vulnerable women and populations where there is poverty, deprivation, and diversity of ethnic groups. Power is achieved by strengthening the individual power of women and their families, and by the authority that knowing women as individuals and understanding their needs, gives to midwives. Personal power for the woman and the midwife is increased by supporting the development of relationships between childbearing woman and midwives and developing a supportive culture and structure of care. Midwives by virtue of their professional status and expertise hold the potential of power over women. If they are able, rather, to work in the best interests of or 'for' women, an ethical relationship of care, both become empowered. It is working for the woman by knowing her and responding to her needs that authorizes the midwife. Pairman (2006) illustrates this principle in the recorded interviews with midwives working in New Zealand. The description of the relationship of a partnership in this context is apt.

The idea of transformative change in an organization mirrors the transformation of the woman as she becomes a mother. This is a fundamental change in role, a transition that requires new behaviours and skills and ways of seeing the world. Effective midwifery supports the woman to feel powerful as a mother, and the family to hold the personal power to care for the child. This idea of personal power reflects back to the idea of recognizing the parent's central and active role in caring for the baby until adulthood (Page 1989). The parent's sense of personal power is enhanced when the midwife is aware of the importance of the love and commitment of parents to the child for survival and reaching their full potential (Redshaw 2006). Effective midwifery support means respecting the personal autonomy of the woman, and trusting her to make the best decisions for her and her baby and family with the support of family, friends and professionals.

Transformation is a particularly important idea in midwifery because a central concern of transformation is to help to make the purpose and meaning of work clear. The context of midwifery in many parts of the industrialized world is on the conveyer belt of busy acute care hospitals. Evidence of inflexible and uncaring services (DOH 1993) was fundamental to the need for the changes proposed by *Changing Childbirth*. Other specific problems of maternity services in much of the industrialized world, high intervention rates, postnatal depression and low breastfeeding rates may be related to a lack of support of women by midwives.

Developing a positive culture and reviewing purpose

All organizations tend to develop routines and rules that become self-serving to those working in them, for example bringing all women into hospital-based clinics to save staff having to go out into the community, rather than meeting the needs of the people who should be served. This tendency is more pronounced in public service organizations where failure to meet the core needs of the organization will not automatically result in the failure of a business to survive. The organization can easily go off the tracks if it is not intentionally steered to meet the central purpose. 'Organizational transformation requires a review of purpose, and in meeting this newly defined purpose people working within the organization find new ways of doing things' (Beckhard, as cited in Page et al 1995, p. 77). Beckhard goes on to suggest that 'transformation of an organization requires fundamental change at every level, of relationships between people, of employment practices, often of the structure of the organization'. Transformation also involves commitment to a set of values, expressed through practices.

The idea of reviewing the central purpose then, is important in all organizations, but this has been more complex in maternity services where societal changes, such as the emancipation of women and feminism, and more consumer oriented approaches may be seen reflected in the public and consumer voices that let us know that 'all was not well with the maternity Services' (House of Commons 1992). This discontent, given that mortality rates were lower than they had ever been, was difficult for many to understand and seemed paradoxical.

Culture of care is an expression of centrally held values in an organization. *Changing Childbirth* (DOH 1993) described what is known as 'woman-centred care' and House of Commons (1992) spoke of putting women 'central stage'. These concepts have continued to be a part of new government policy in England (DOH 2004). Organizations should be clear whom they are meant to be serving, and what their service is. Woman-centred care requires that we focus on the needs of woman while supporting staff to serve those women. The process of reviewing purpose and values in the establishment of one-to-one midwifery is described in some detail (Page et al 1995). This clarification of values and purpose may be somewhat easier when a service is being restructured and staff will be recruited to join a new service, but the process can and should be as effective in more traditional standard organizations (Page 2003a). The idea of clarifying purpose is also important to changing the structure of care. Many innovations were developed over the last decades that were said to be aimed at improving continuity of care, while setting up a large team of midwives which could never achieve continuity of care.

BEING A MIDWIFE TO MIDWIVES – SPEAKING FROM EXPERIENCE

As well as restructuring to enable continuity of care and transforming the service to create a positive culture it is also important to ensure efficiency and smooth running. There are practical steps that need to be taken.

There are a number of ways to change maternity services so that midwives may practice more effectively and sensitively, including a shift to primary care, the development of birth centres, and rebuilding premises. Much of my work over 20 years has been in transforming large established maternity services that encompass community and hospital, both by developing continuity of care schemes, but also by leading transformative change. The good or functional service described in the introduction serves women and supports positive childbirth, providing woman-centred services. It does this in large part by supporting staff, including midwives, to do their best. A good maternity service will give staff the opportunity to practice fully, learn, grow and develop, and generally find work enjoyable and challenging.

In the remainder of this chapter I will describe practical steps that may be taken in the process of transformation. There is something of a caution here though. While the steps may seem practical and simple, the politics, relationship building, and reorganization required, are based on complex processes that need to be understood. Just

as midwives and researchers need education, training, support and development for their role so do leaders and managers.

To take on this challenge of transformative and practical change, particularly when the service is dysfunctional, can be extremely difficult, tiring and sometimes distressing. Maternity services that are dysfunctional do great harm not only to those being cared for but also to staff working in them. While transformative and practice changes are led on an analytical understanding of what is happening, and what may help, many of the steps are practical, and will work over time. This last part of the chapter is intended to give practical advice.

Where to start – gain personal support

Often transformational change requires working on a number of areas and levels at once. The start of such work can be exciting, but also daunting. It is important to remember that dysfunction and function run in cycles. Once a cycle is broken it may reverse apparently quickly, in either direction. The first step is to gain personal support. Transformational change requires deep involvement. A mentor outside of the organization will help keep a sense of perspective. Everyone has his or her blind spots. Talking through and being encouraged to think about what is happening is crucial. A good starting point is being clear on personal values and goals but also in clarifying the goals of the organization. Every aspect of change, and decision on priorities, needs to be informed by these values and principles.

Developing of visible leadership

One of the themes that comes through the research on why midwives leave and why they stay is the separation between midwives and their managers. I always feel concerned when I hear midwives talk about 'the management'; it is indicative of real alienation. It is often as though they inhabit different worlds, and in some sense they do. Managers, particularly those in middle management, often have to translate the goals of the layer above them into operation, and often this is difficult, as in for example, making cost savings. They also bridge the divide in highly complex organizations in which change is constant, and there are huge amounts of information to understand, process and channel. The nature of work in most modern health services is dictated by many meetings, multifaceted accountability, and hoards of information as well as communication by electronic and internet communications. Yet managers and leaders need to be visible, to understand the work and needs of the midwives they lead, and to help them resolve their problems. It is a priority therefore for mangers to be seen, to walk about, to talk to staff, and where possible, to continue to practice. Managers need to be available when problems occur that need their support, and to contain anxiety.

Developing systems of support for professionals

Support for midwives often parallels the support needed by women. Support includes information, discussion, ongoing training and education not only to allow the job to be done, but to help understand what is going on in the health service as a whole. This is particularly important in a service like the National Health Service that is bureaucratic by nature (Deery and Kirkham 2006). Deery (1999) recommends that systems such as clinical supervision which integrates reflection, education and personal support may help midwives. The support cannot be one way, just as the relationship between women and their midwives is at its best reciprocal, so must the relationship between midwives and their managers be reciprocal. Kirkham and Stapleton describe the need for managers and leaders to involve midwives themselves in understanding the problems they face and to involve them in the difficult work of resolution (2001, 2004).

Developing interdisciplinary work and role clarification

Midwives work in the context of complex services that are intended to provide women with specialist support when it is needed. Safe services provide an interface in which midwives may refer the women they are caring for to specialist support, while having their expertise acknowledged and respected. However, it is important that all staff are clear about their roles, their

unique functions. All staff hold the same aim, to ensure that the outcomes of pregnancy birth and the early weeks of life are healthy and positive. While there is some overlap, midwives, doctors, doulas and nurses have different roles in reaching these aims. Joint work in education, research, training and team development will enhance relationships, but differences need to be understood and respected.

Break down hierarchies

The work of Menzies (1988) illustrates the way hierarchies function to separate midwives not only from the women they care for, but also separate staff from each other, and midwives from their managers. A hierarchy forms a chain of command in which those higher up the chain have little practical understanding of the world that those operating in practice inhabit. Those at the top pass down information and instructions, making decisions a long way from the place of practice. Virtual parallel universes develop in hierarchical organizations. To break down a hierarchy means to give those near the place of practice as much autonomy as possible, while providing a clear framework of principles, values, aims and objectives for them to operate in. Breaking down a hierarchy includes the need to develop flatter management structures, with a focus on team building and value clarification, and the development of clear goals. The majority of managerial roles in midwifery should include direct involvement in clinical practice.

Consciously developing ethical leadership

Leaders and managers of services, as well as the staff working at grass roots level, face ethical dilemmas not only in relation to clinical care but also in relation to management of staff. Consider the dilemmas of the mentor who likes a student or the return to practice midwife, but needs to fail her on an assessment or the colleague whose standards of practice are not good, and needs to be reported. Clearly, the needs of women and families who are entrusted to our care always need to come first, but these situations can be difficult and challenging. For managers who are involved in investigating complaints of poor practice or bullying it is important that while the needs of women and families are paramount that natural principles of justice are understood. Most large organizations now will have human resource guidelines and support; nevertheless there is still the need for individual judgement, and a commitment to fair processes. The work of Kirkham and Stapleton (2001, 2004) and others describes midwifery organizations that are unsupportive and often contain bullying. Clear messages about bullying behaviour being unacceptable are required. Often those who have been involved in bullying need extensive support, and may well be helped to develop more functional relationships. In a service where relationships are valued, all training, education, communications must focus on building positive relationships and communications, and provide models of positive relationships in action by leaders within the service.

Reviewing resources

No matter how strong the leadership, inadequate resources, not enough midwives, computer systems that don't work or are too complex and inadequate support for midwives, will make the development of a functioning service more difficult. Midwifery is extremely, pardon the pun, labour intensive and forms a large part of the budget. The articulation and measurement of the need for more resources, with the ability to manage them carefully is often a large part of the management of maternity services where midwives are employed by the service. It should be mentioned here that continuity of care or caseload models are far more cost effective than fragmented models (Piercy 1996).

Environmental change

A few years ago many maternity services in England were provided with extra money from the government to rebuild or update their buildings. This physical change often brought about a change in practice. Even without a lot of money the provision of inexpensive furniture or props for women to be more comfortable will help. Redecorating and tidying may give a renewed sense of purpose. The NCT has a toolkit that will help in assessing the physical environment. Attention to the physical environment is important to women (Page 2006b) and to midwives.

Magic in the intention

Once when I was visiting a government department in Canada as a part of a team who were working to have midwifery integrated into the health service, we were prepared by a coach who, at the end of the briefing, told us to remember that 'there is magic in the intention'. These words have always stayed with me. By consciously thinking about and imagining what you want to achieve, it seems that work and discussions, even in what may seem like impossible situations, are more successful.

Room for this conscious imaginative and creative work is crucial, and remembering what it is you want to achieve is very powerful.

When setting up one of the first team midwifery projects in the UK, an extremely difficult task, I was about to give up, when I talked to a woman who had been cared for by a midwife she knew. Her words, that were very simple but that described the essence of what was important, kept me going. Even now when I get tired I will find it is often the words of women, or a midwife who has found her niche, that will help restore my energy.

I hope this chapter will contribute to an understanding of why maternity services often stop midwives from practising good midwifery, and will help inform the work of making the maternity services a place where midwives 'may be the midwives they want to be' (Curtis, Ball and Kirkham 2006).

To support midwives to support women, to be a midwife to midwifery, is to support the passageway to life, the birth of the baby, and the birth of the mother and family. This support of midwives to be effective and sensitive to the needs of women and families in their care will reverberate into healthier families, and a better, kinder world. Transforming midwifery services is a step to transforming society. The work of midwifery is of the utmost importance to all and should be celebrated, treasured, nurtured and developed with the commitment, knowledge and skill it deserves.

Summary Box: Empowering the midwives

- Restructure at least part of the service to develop continuity of care, but also transform the organization as a whole.
- Gain personal support.
- Develop visible leadership.
- Develop systems of support for professionals and professional development and education – break down hierarchies.

- Develop interdisciplinary work and role clarification.
- Develop consciously just and ethical leadership and standards of behaviour, communication and practice.
- Review resources.
- Make environmental change.

References

Association of Radical Midwives 1986 The Vision: Proposals for the future of the maternity services. ARM, Ormskirk.

Barclay L, Jones L 1996 Midwifery trends and practice in Australia. Churchill Livingstone, Australia.

Brodie P 1996 Being with women: The experiences of Australian team midwives. Unpublished master's of nursing dissertation University of Technology Sydney, Sydney, Australia.

Chapple J 2006 Achieving better outcomes of maternity services: the role of public health. In: LA Page, R McCandlish (Eds). The new midwifery: Science and sensitivity in practice. Churchill Livingstone, Edinburgh, pp. 291–310.

Curtis P, Ball L, Kirkham M 2006 Why do midwives leave? (Not) being the midwife you want to be. British Journal of Midwifery 14(1): 27–31.

Davis-Floyd R 2001 The technocratic, humanistic, and holistic paradigms of childbirth. International Journal of Gynaecology and Obstetrics, (Special Edition) 75: S5–S23.

Deery R 1999 Improving relationships through clinical supervision: 2. British Journal of Midwifery 7(4): 251–254.

Deery R, Kirkham M 2006 Supporting midwives to support women. In: LA Page, R McCandlish (Eds). The new midwifery: Science and sensitivity in practice. Churchill Livingstone, Edinburgh, pp. 125–140.

Department of Health 1993 Changing childbirth: Part 1. Report of the Expert Maternity Group. HMSO, London.

Department of Health and Department for Education and Skills 2004 National Service Framework for children, young people and maternity service: The Maternity Standard. DH publications, London.

Dunkley-Bent J 2006 Reducing inequalities in childbirth: the midwife's role in public health. In: LA Page, R McCandlish (Eds). The new midwifery: Science and sensitivity in practice. Churchill Livingstone, Edinburgh, pp. 311–332.

Flint C, Poulengeris P 1987 The Know Your Midwife Report, Pub 49. London SE26 6RZ.

Freeley M 1995 Team midwifery – A personal experience. In: LA Page (Ed). Effective group practice in midwifery: Working with women. Blackwell Science, Oxford, pp. 3–11.

Haggerty J, Reid RJ and Freeman GKI 2003 Continuity of care: A multidisciplinary review. British Medical Journal 327: 1219–1221.

House of Commons 1992 Health Committee Second Report on The Maternity Services to the House of Commons. HMSO, London.

House of Commons 2003a Health Committee Report. Fourth report of session 2002–2003. Provision of maternity services, volumes 1 and 2. HC, London.

House of Commons 2003b Health Committee Report. Eighth report of session 2002–2003. Inequalities in access to services, volumes 1 and 2. HC, London.

House of Commons 2003c Health Committee Report. Ninth report of session 2002–2003. Choice in Maternity Services, volumes 1 and 2. HC, London.

Hunt S, Symonds A 1995 The social meaning of midwifery. Macmillan Press, Basingstoke.

Kirkham M, Stapleton H 2001 Midwives support needs as childbirth changes. MIDIRS Midwifery Digest 11: 157–163.

Kirkham M, Stapleton H 2004 The culture of the maternity services in Wales and England as a barrier to informed choice. In: M Kirkham (Ed). Informed choice in maternity care. Palgrave Macmillan, Basingstoke, pp. 117–145.

Menzies I 1988 Containing anxiety in institutions. Selected Essays 1. Free Association Books, London.

McCourt C, Hirst J, Page LA 2000 Dimensions and attributes of caring: Women's perceptions. In: LA Page (Ed). The new midwifery: Science and sensitivity in practice. Churchill Livingstone, Edinburgh, pp. 269–287.

McCourt C, Stevens T, Sandall J, Brodie P 2006 Working with women: Developing continuity of carer in practice. In: LA Page, R McCandlish (Eds). The new midwifery: Science and sensitivity in practice. Churchill Livingstone, Edinburgh, pp. 141–166.

Page LA 1989 The midwife's role in modern health care. In: S Kitzinger (Ed). The midwife challenge. Pandora Press, Seattle, pp. 251–260.

Page L, Bentley R, Jones 1995 Transforming the organization. In: L Page (Ed). Effective group practice in midwifery: Working with women. Blackwell Science, Oxford, pp. 77–94.

Page LA 2003a Woman-centred and midwife friendly care: Principles and practice. In: D Fraser (Ed). Myles textbook for midwives. Churchill Livingstone, Edinburgh, pp. 31–47.

Page LA 2003b One-to-one midwifery: Restoring the 'with woman' relationship in midwifery. Journal of Midwifery and Women's Health 48(2): 119–125.

Page LA 2004 Working with women in childbirth. Unpublished PhD thesis, University of Technology Sydney, Sydney.

Page LA 2006b An ideal birth environment? The right facilities and support for women. British Journal of Midwifery 14: 46.

Page LA, McCandlish R 2006 Introduction. In: LA Page, R McCandlish (Eds). The new midwifery: Science and sensitivity in practice. Churchill Livingstone, Edinburgh, pp. xiii–xx.

Pairman S 2006 Midwifery partnership: Working with women. In: LA Page, R McAndlish (Eds). The new midwifery: Science and sensitivity in practice. Churchill Livingstone, Edinburgh, pp. 73–96.

Piercy J, Page LA, McCourt C 1996 Economic study. In: C McCourt, LA Page (Eds). Report on the evaluation of one-to-one midwifery. Thames Valley University, London, pp. 14–23.

Redshaw M 2006 First relationships and the growth of love and commitment. In: LA Page, R McCandlish (Eds). The new midwifery: Science and sensitivity in practice. Churchill Livingstone, Edinburgh, pp. 21–48.

Robinson S 1989 The role of the midwife: Opportunities and constraints. In: I Chalmers, M Enkin, MJNC Kierse (Eds). Effective care in pregnancy and childbirth. Oxford University Press, Oxford, pp. 162–189.

Sandall J 1997 Midwives burn out and continuity of care. British Journal of Midwifery, 5:106–111.

Saultz JW 2003 Defining and measuring interpersonal continuity of care. Annals of Family Medicine 1(3): 134–143.

Stevens TA 2003 Midwife to mid wif: A study of caseload midwifery. Unpublished doctoral thesis, Thames Valley University, London.

Seccombe I, Stock J 1995 Team midwifery. In: L Page (Ed). Effective group practice in midwifery: Working with women. Blackwell Science, Oxford, pp. 106–116.

Weatherston LA 1985 Midwifery in the hospital: A team approach to perinatal care. Dimensions in Health Service 62: 15–16 & 22.

Chapter **9**

Birth territory: The besieged territory of the obstetrician

Michel Odent

INTRODUCTION

This chapter begins by establishing that there are only two obligatory characters in the childbirth drama: the mother and the baby. That is why any interpretation of the unstable relationship between obstetricians, midwives, and other caregivers must be preceded by an overview of the basic needs of labouring women and newborn babies. Our current understanding of birth physiology is based on the adrenaline–oxytocin antagonism and on the inhibitory effects of neocortical activity on the process of parturition. This leads us to understand that a labouring woman needs to feel secure, without feeling observed, in a warm enough place, and to be protected against any sort of neocortical stimulation (language, light, lack of privacy, being aware of a possible danger, etc). I then provide an historical overview of how the birth territory came to be the domain of the obstetrician in Europe, and describe how that process is being undermined by newly developing specialties such as sonography, fetal medicine, obstetric anesthesiology, neonatology, perinatology, epidemiology, and genetic counselling; it is also undermined by the health needs of older and chronically ill women who in the past would never have become pregnant in the first place. The chapter concludes by bringing us back to the current global situation and by looking towards the future. The focus on the physiology of childbirth and the two main actors must be the basis of both authentic obstetrics and authentic midwifery. In this way we will create situations that enable as many women as possible to give birth thanks to the release of a complex 'cocktail of love hormones'. The future of humanity is at stake.

WHOSE TERRITORY? CENTRE STAGE: MOTHER AND BABY

Before considering the 'territory' of the obstetrician, in relation to the 'territory' of other possible persons involved in pregnancy and childbirth, we must first recall that, whatever the geographical and historical contexts, childbirth has only two obligatory actors: the mother and the baby. This is why we must first refer to the basic needs of labouring women and newborn babies. Physiologists offer a reference point from which we should try not to deviate too much. While all societies have interfered in the birth process, mostly via beliefs and rituals, physiologists study what is universal and cross-cultural. After thousands of years of culturally controlled childbirth, their perspective is the only one that can lead us to re-discover the basic needs of birthing women and newborn babies. An overview of birth physiology will help us to interpret the unstable relationship between obstetricians, midwives and other health professionals.

Three basic needs to be met (safety, privacy and warmth)

Our understanding of birth physiology is based on one simple fact we must constantly refer to. It is that adrenaline and oxytocin are antagonistic. Adrenaline is the hormone mammals release in emergency situations, particularly when they are scared, cold or feel observed. Oxytocin is the key hormone of parturition because of both its mechanical effects (inducing and maintaining effective uterine contractions), and its behavioural effects as the typical 'love hormone'. Mammals cannot release oxytocin when their level of adrenaline is high. Since humans are mammals, we may conclude from the physiological perspective that a woman in labour needs to feel secure, without feeling observed, and she needs to be in a warm enough environment.

Preventing neocortical stimulation

While the physiological perspective can easily identify the basic needs of labouring women, it can also make easily understood the specifically human handicaps in the period surrounding birth. The human handicaps are related to the huge development of that part of the brain called the neocortex, which can be presented as the brain of the intellect, or the thinking brain. It is thanks to our highly developed neocortex that we can talk, count and be logical and rational. When there are inhibitions – during the birth process or during any sort of sexual experience – they originate in the neocortex.

Nature found a solution to overcoming this human handicap in the period surrounding birth. The neocortex is supposed to be at rest so that primitive brain structures (hypothalamus, pituitary gland) can more easily release the necessary hormones. It is well-known that women who give birth tend to cut themselves off from our world, to forget what they have read or been taught; they dare to do what a civilized woman would never dare to do in her daily social life (daring to scream, to swear, etc.); they can find themselves in the most unexpected, often quadrupedal posture. I have heard women saying afterwards: 'I was on another planet'. When a labouring woman is 'on another planet', this means that the activity of her neocortex is reduced.

This essential aspect of human birth physiology implies that one of the basic needs of labouring women is to be protected against any sort of neocortical stimulation. From a practical point of view it is useful to explain what this means and to review the well-known factors that can stimulate the human neocortex.

Language and silence

Language, particularly rational language is one such factor. When we communicate with language we process what we perceive with our neocortex. This implies, for example, that if there is a birth attendant, one of her main qualities is her capacity to keep a low profile, to remain silent, and to avoid, in particular, asking precise questions. Although it is apparently simple, it will probably take a long time to rediscover the importance of silence.

Bright light

Bright light is another factor that stimulates the human neocortex. Electroencephalographers know that the trace exploring brain activity can be influenced by visual stimulation. We usually close the curtains and switch off the lights when we want to reduce the activity of our intellect in order to go to sleep. This implies that, from a physiological perspective, a dim light should in general facilitate the birth process. It will also take a long time to convince many health professionals that this is a serious issue. It is noticeable that as soon as a labouring woman is on 'another planet' she is spontaneously driven towards postures that tend to protect her against all sorts of visual stimulation. For example, she may be on her hands and knees, as if praying. Apart from reducing back pain, this common posture has many positive effects, such as eliminating the main reason for fetal distress (no compression of the big vessels that run along the spine) and facilitating optimal rotation of the baby's body.

Feeling observed and the need for privacy and to feel secure

A feeling of being observed can also be presented as another type of neocortical stimulation. The physiological response to the presence of an observer has been scientifically studied. In fact, it is common knowledge that we all feel different when we know we are being observed. In other words, privacy is a factor that facilitates the reduction of neocortical control. It is ironic that all non-human mammals, whose neocortex is not as developed as ours, have a strategy for giving birth in privacy – those who are normally active during the night, like rats, tend to give birth during the day, and conversely, others like horses, who are active during the day, tend to give birth at night. Wild goats give birth in the most inaccessible mountain areas. Our close relatives, the chimpanzees, also move away from the group. The importance of privacy implies, for example, that there is a difference between the attitude of a midwife staying in front of a woman in labour and watching her, and another one just sitting in a corner. It implies also that we should be reluctant to introduce any device that can be perceived as a way to observe the woman,

Box 9.1   Questions for discussion

- How do you reduce neocortical stimulation with birthing women?
- Have you considered your own presence in the space with the woman?
- What is the lighting like?
- How warm is the room?

may it be a video camera or an electronic fetal monitor.

Any situation associated with a release of adrenaline also implies a stimulation of the neocortex. When there is a possible danger, it is an advantage to be alert and attentive. This is another way to explain the need to feel secure.

The importance of the third stage of labour and the oxytocin peak

The physiological perspective leads us also to focus on the key event that occurs during the 'third stage of labour', which is between the birth of the baby and the delivery of the placenta. This key event is the release of a high peak of oxytocin. One can even claim, referring to Swedish studies (Nissen 1995), that the highest peak of oxytocin a woman can reach during her whole life is immediately after the birth of her baby; higher than for the birth itself; than during an orgasm; than during a milk ejection reflex; higher than during any situation associated with a release of this hormone. As in any other circumstances, this oxytocin release is highly dependent on environmental factors. In the particular case of the third stage of labour the first important environmental factors are related to the ambient temperature. The surroundings must be very warm as soon as the baby is born. Mothers never complain that it is too hot just after the birth of the baby. If they are shivering, it is because the place is not warm enough. Another condition is that the mother, who is still 'on another planet', is not distracted at all and has nothing else to do than to feel the contact with the baby's skin, to look at the baby's eyes, and to smell the baby.

The release of a high peak of oxytocin, just after the birth itself, is vital for several reasons. First it is necessary for an easy and fast delivery

---

Box 9.2 Questions for discussion

- How am I going to improve behavioural oxytocin release for women in third stage?
- Is this stage really so important?
- Have you ever thought about the way the future of the infant's relationships are created in this moment when mother and baby meet?
- What effect will it have on the mother and baby if I keep mother and baby together immediately after birth; facilitate undisturbed skin to skin touching between mother and baby; enable a physiological third stage; avoid routine suctioning of the baby; dry the baby gently; provide warmth from blankets laid over the pair, avoid speaking and interrupting the relationship; delay weighing and measuring activities; let parents discover the sex of the baby in their own time?
- Is there a physiological need for a third person to be present at birth?

Box 9.3 Questions for discussion

- Who do you think needs to be present with the birthing woman?
- Her mother?
- Someone in the role of mother?
- Could this mother role be assumed by the midwife?
- How comfortable are you in the role of mother?
- How do you be 'present' to someone in labour in your practice and avoid being perceived as judging or observing?

---

of the placenta, without any dangerous blood loss. Furthermore oxytocin has behavioural effects and is now considered as the main 'hormone of love'.

The physiological perspective leads to the conclusion that the presence at birth of a 'third person' (apart from mother and baby) cannot be considered a basic need. The basic needs are privacy and the need to feel secure. Similar conclusions may be drawn from cross-cultural studies. We must keep in mind that the concept of birth attendant is probably more recent than commonly believed. Films of life and childbirth among the Eipos in New Guinea (Schiefenhovel 1978), written documents about pre-agricultural societies such as, for example, the Kung San (Eaton 1998), and word-of-mouth reports from Amazonian ethnic groups suggest that there has been a phase in the history of humanity when women used to isolate themselves when giving birth, like all mammals. However midwifery is such a widespread and deep-rooted concept that we cannot study the 'territory' of the medical man without referring to the 'third person'. Once more we must resort to the physiological perspective to interpret the reason for midwifery and the specific role of the midwife.

It seems that all over the world and through the ages, women always had a tendency to give birth close to their mother, or close to a substitute for their mother – an experienced mother or grandmother – in the framework of the extended family or in the framework of the community. The midwife was originally a mother figure. In an ideal world, our mother is the prototype of the person with whom one feels secure, without feeling observed and judged. She is the prototype of the person intended to offer protection. The privacy of the birthing woman needs to be protected, in particular against the curiosity of occasional wandering men, so conditions for an irresistible 'fetus ejection reflex' are met (Odent 1987). Birth physiology is usually looked at from a purely pelvic perspective. This is why it is commonplace to claim that the main role of the midwife was originally to overcome mechanical problems.

After making clear the basic needs of the two obligatory actors and the original reason for the 'third person', we are in a position to explore the 'territory' of the obstetrician. The territory of the obstetrician and his ancestors is so vague and so unstable that we'll start from the historical perspective in order to analyse the current situation and to look towards the future.

THE TERRITORY OF THE OBSTETRICIAN BEFORE THE NINETEENTH CENTURY

We must first clarify our definition of the word 'territory'. Terms such as territory, domain, sphere, province, field, scope, realm, room, and area imply the concept of limits. All of them may be understood in a literal, purely spatial sense. All of them may also be understood in a figurative sense, referring to limits in terms of competence, role, interest and activities. We will consider both the literal and figurative meanings. We must also clarify our definition of the word 'obstetrician', which did not appear in England until the middle of the nineteenth century, when several distinguished 'obstetricians' were raised to the dignity of 'Fellows of the College of Physicians'. We must include in our definition the ancestors of the modern obstetricians: shaman, medical man, man–midwife, barber, surgeon, surgeon–apothecary, physician.

Before the nineteenth century any question about the personal 'spatial territory' of the obstetrician was irrelevant. The ancestors of the modern obstetricians, whatever their names, had no personal space at their disposal. Women were giving birth on their own 'territory'. Women always had a tendency to protect the birthing place against the presence of men, particularly the medical men. Many women had such strong objections to male attendance that during the sixteenth century, in Hamburg, a doctor was condemned to death and burnt alive after disguising himself as a woman in order to see a birth. At that time, it was said, women were prepared to die rather than admit a man to the lying-in room (Von Siebold 1839).

OBSTETRICIANS, INSTRUMENTS AND LITERACY

Although, in most societies we know about, childbirth was 'women's business', this is not to say that male physicians never interested themselves in childbirth. Male physicians have often been attributed two spheres of competence. The first sphere of competence was to intervene in desperate situations when called by the midwives. Before the invention of the forceps, all the medical man could do was usually to remove the infant piece-meal by use of hooks and perforators, or, if there was still hope of delivering a living child, to perform a caesarean section on the body of the mother after her death (Donnison 1977). The realm of instruments is eminently male. The second sphere of competence of literate male physicians has been to write about childbirth, mainly for the purpose of educating midwives and of instructing the other physicians on how to supervise women delivering babies. Hippocrates, Aristotle, Celsus, Galen, Soranus of Ephesus and other writers on medical matters devoted part of their works to the subject. The realm of books is also originally eminently male.

The point is that since the medical man was called in for disasters only, he had little opportunity of gaining a real understanding of the birth process and of the basic needs of labouring women. However, the main ambition of many physicians was to control the education of midwives. It is significant that, for more than a century, the Chamberlens considered the use of their forceps a precious family secret. Their objective was to be recognized as the best 'obstetricians', so that they would deserve to monopolize the education of midwives. At that time, the expanding sphere of competence of the physicians was already a threat for the autonomy of midwives. In Western Europe this autonomy was also threatened by the Church, which used to control the selection of women who would become midwives. The territory of midwives was besieged.

Forceps establish the authority and the territory of the obstetrician

History can help us in interpreting the deep-rooted and widespread lack of understanding of birth physiology. It is the introduction of the forceps at the beginning of the eighteenth century that precipitated the history of rivalry between midwives and medical men and prepared the turning point of the nineteenth century. Forceps enabled the medical man to deliver live infants in cases where previously either child or mother or both would have died, and also to shorten tedious labours. Furthermore it happened that medical men accepted being in attendance for routine cases, placing themselves in direct competition with the midwives and gaining a hold on the greater part of the best-paid midwifery. At the same phase of history, lying-in hospitals appeared and developed. The Paris Hotel-Dieu played an important role in the training of French midwives. This role was so widely recognized that a lying-in hospital was founded in Dublin. Similar establishments followed in London and in Edinburgh. Although such lying-hospitals may be considered the precursors of modern maternity hospitals, maternity units and departments of obstetrics, it is noticeable that originally they remained the territory of midwives. The Head Midwife at the Hotel-Dieu was independent of the medical staff and used to call the surgeon only when she considered instruments were necessary. French and British lying-hospitals took no male students. Midwives were also in charge of normal births in the early 20th century in New Zealand with the advent of the St Helen's Hospitals in 1905 (set up for wives of working class men). St Helen's Hospitals were staffed solely by midwives with a medical superintendent who could be called in when the midwife identified the need for one. Originally these hospitals would not allow the training of medical students (Wood and Foureur 2005).

AFTER THE NINETEENTH CENTURY TURNING POINT

There are many reasons why the middle of the nineteenth century should be considered a turning point in the history of the relationship between midwifery and medicine. First, it is the time when 'obstetricians' became respected physicians. In England, the College of Physicians accepted some of them as its 'Fellows'. Second, the practice of midwifery was regulated with the backing of physicians and surgeons. In England, the College of Surgeons set up a Midwifery Licence, while in Paris it was established via a decree that, after being qualified by a 'Faculté de Médecine', the so-called first-class 'sages-femmes' could practice everywhere in France. Another influential reason for the turning point is that the prestigious departments of obstetrics and gynaecology of the Humboldt-Universitat, in Berlin, of the Allgemeines Frankenhaus, in Wien (Vienna), and of 'La Maternité Port-Royal', in Paris, attracted world famous practitioners.

Within a few years there were spectacular technical advances. James Young Simpson, the outstanding obstetrician from Edinburgh, discovered the anaesthetic qualities of chloroform and championed obstetric anaesthesia. The famous forceps he presented in 1848 are still in use all over the world, although at least 600 obstetric forceps have since been described in detail (Bordahl 1998). The influence of Semmelweis in Wien,

and Lister in England, led to the concept of antisepsis and opened a new era in the history of gynaecologic surgery.

One of the effects of this cascade of technical advances was to clarify the roles of midwives and obstetricians. Dr James Edmunds, from London, an early disciple of Semmelweis, who had performed one of the first successful caesarean operations, expressed his point of view without any ambiguity. According to him, all ordinary cases should be handed over to well-instructed midwives of good education who would call in 'well-known obstetricians' when there was difficulty or danger (Edmunds 1986). Edmund's opinion was that it was important to spare 'delicate-minded' women the 'ordeal' of male attendance.

During this phase of fast technological advances, there was no open rivalry between the midwives and the pure specialized obstetricians of big cities such as Berlin, Wien, Paris, London, Edinburgh and Dublin. Outstanding obstetricians of that time were focused on developing new techniques and instruments, and were not interested in the evolving relationship between midwifery and obstetrics. Their main tacit ambition was often to attach their name to an instrument. It is thanks to their forceps, that the names of Simpson, Elliott and Tarnier are transmitted from generation to generation. It is thanks to his fetal stethoscope that the name of Pinard is well known. The rivalry was much more between midwives and general practitioners. Far from wishing to see midwives trained and regulated, many physicians looked forward to the day when midwives could be legally excluded from practice. In affluent areas of big cities such as the West End of London, physicians took control of the majority of births. Physicians also took control of birth in the New World (the colonies of Britain): Australia, New Zealand and North America.

Rivalries between physicians and midwives did not take the same directions in Europe and in North America. In Europe, endless discussions led to regulation of midwifery practice. In continental Europe, most countries took the most important steps before the end of the nineteenth century. In England, after decades of almost non-stop controversy within the medical profession, the 1902 Midwives Act received Royal Assent. Interestingly, the Act did not specify that a majority of members of the Midwives board (in charge of the registration of midwives) should be medical practitioners. The 1902 Act was completed in 1936 by another act, recommending that midwives should send abnormal cases to hospital, instead of calling a physician. In the pre-war context it was already clear that in many areas general practitioners lacked that experience of attending normal labours, which is a necessary preliminary to the understanding of abnormal cases. Latent rivalries were mostly between general practitioners and more specialized physicians.

In the USA, on the other hand, midwives had already virtually disappeared at the beginning of the twentieth century. Doctors had already gained a grip on the birth process and the status and role of the midwife were dwindling with equal rapidity. Midwifery was already associated with so-called ignorant, illiterate immigrant women. There was no question of providing them with adequate training. The elimination of midwives was undoubtedly a consequence of a deep-rooted quasi-cultural lack of understanding of the basic needs of birthing women. That is why it was easily accepted and even welcomed by the greatest part of the American population. Physician care was presented in terms of better care: we must keep in mind that a century ago, in the USA, the risk of dying from pregnancy or childbirth was around 400 per 100,000. There were also economic reasons. Not only was the volume of business for physicians limited by midwives, but since midwives' clients were mostly poor, the 'clinical material' with which to train new generations of obstetricians was diminished as well. In such a context, hospitalization became more widespread earlier than in Europe, and a famous American professor of obstetrics, Joseph DeLee, could become highly influential. He was the author of several obstetrical textbooks, a sought-after speaker, and the inventor or modifier of many obstetrical tools. In his famous 1920 article and speech to fellow obstetricians entitled 'the prophylactic use of forceps', he noted that 'labor is a pathological process'. He recommended the routine use of forceps and episiotomy at every birth. He suggested that the 'patient' should be sedated and that ether should be given when the fetus entered the birth canal; ergot or a similar agent used to hasten the delivery of the placenta which would then be extracted with a 'shoehorn maneuver'. DeLee's treatise was so influential in America, that by the 1930s 'prophylactic obstetrics' had become the norm.

It was also around the turn of the century that work had begun, in Germany, on the effects of a mixture of drugs, morphine and scopolamine. Several American women were so excited by the prospect of a completely painless delivery that they went to Freiburg, Germany, during the opening months of World War 1. They returned to promote 'Twilight Sleep'. The technique involved injecting the woman with morphine at the beginning of labour and then giving her a dose of the amnesic drug scopolamine, which caused her to forget what was happening. During the second stage the doctor gave ether or chloroform. The campaign for Twilight Sleep was so successful that it attracted women to hospitals and at the same time made them more manageable during labour and delivery and allowed use of other techniques. The concept of prophylactic obstetrics promoted by Joseph DeLee, associated with the popularity of Twilight Sleep, explain the reasons for the 'territory' of the American specialized obstetricians rapidly becoming larger than ever. Their territory in obstetrical units was threatened neither by the submissive nurses, other physicians, the sedated 'patients', nor by the excluded father.

The divergence between the histories of childbirth on both sides of the Atlantic Ocean deepened further during the Second World War. With the discovery of the antibacterial effects of sulphonamides in the late 1930s, the use of penicillin, which began in the 1940s, and at the same time the development of blood transfusion, American women had further reasons to place themselves in the hands of specialized obstetricians when giving birth. At the same time, in Europe, most doctors were serving in the armies and midwives became more autonomous than ever. It is significant, for example, that the great autonomy Dutch midwives still have today is to a certain extent a consequence of regulations established during the war. Furthermore, immediately after the war, there was a fast evolution towards socialized medicine in Europe, but not in the USA. The British National Health Service became reality in 1948, while the French 'Sécurité Sociale' was officially created in 1946. In spite of inevitable differences between large cities and rural areas, between social classes, and between ethnic groups, we can claim that in the middle of the twentieth century obstetricians had control over childbirth in North America, while in Europe childbirth was still 'women's business'.

ENTERING CONTEMPORARY HISTORY

We penetrate the framework of contemporary history when witnesses are still alive who can furnish evidence of what happened during the investigated period. From my personal viewpoint, I am tempted to claim that the contemporary history of obstetrics started in 1953, when I spent half a year in the 'Hôpital Boucicaut' in Paris as an 'externe'. An 'externe' was a selected medical student with minor responsibility.

Officially, at that time, the maternity unit of a big hospital in a city such as Paris was the territory of the obstetrician. It is significant that in our jargon we would say, for example: 'en ce moment je suis chez Suzor' (I am currently at Suzor's). We were using the name of the obstetrician in charge of the unit (e.g. Suzor) when referring to our current clinical activities. In reality, such a maternity unit was the territory of midwives. If I was given permission to 'deliver' some babies, it was thanks to the goodwill of some midwives. In the case of a difficult birth in the middle of the night, the highly autonomous midwife would call a junior doctor for a forceps delivery. The young doctor had to obey, without discussing the decision taken by the midwife. The chief doctor was often visible between 10 am and noon during the weekdays, when doing a round in the unit or chatting with other members of staff. The rest of the time he was probably taking care of middle-class women who were attracted by small private clinics and who wanted to 'be delivered' by one particular doctor. Rates of home births were already quite low. Outside the big cities there were not many specialized obstetricians. There were independent midwives who occasionally had to call a doctor when a complication occurred. This doctor usually was either a surgeon or a local general practitioner familiar with the use of forceps. In the early 1950s the practice of obstetrics was not considered prestigious. It did not attract the elite of medical students. There were many pejorative sayings about obstetrics being a sort of second-class specialty.

An ascending status – the lower segment caesarean section

It took only two decades for obstetrics to get out of its second-class status and for the obstetrician to significantly enlarge his territory. The cascade of important scientific, technical and conceptual advances that occurred in the 1950s can explain this fast mutation.

The development of the low segmental technique of caesarean is undoubtedly a landmark in the history of childbirth. Although the new safe technique had been described as early as 1926 by Munro Kerr, a professor of midwifery at the University of Glasgow (Kerr 1926) and promulgated before World War II by influential American obstetricians such as Joseph DeLee, it was in the 1950s that it started to routinely supersede the old technique. However there were several obstacles to the rapid development of the new technique. Many obstetricians had a deep-rooted attachment to the forceps, which for three centuries had been the symbol of their discipline. Also, very few doctors involved in childbirth had a surgical background. Obstetricians were reluctant to become dependent on the more prestigious surgeons, who could almost overnight learn the low segmental technique. I was in a position to perceive the semi-conscious motivations of different practitioners, according to their age and their background, at a time when I was trained as a surgeon. I acquired valuable experience of the new technique in 1958 and 1959, while doing my military service in the war of independence in Algeria. In the hospital where I was practising, a caesarean was included in the framework of emergency surgery, like a strangulated hernia or a wounded abdomen on the battlefield.

Oxytocin is synthesized

In 1955, Vincent de Vigneaud discovered how to synthesize the hormone oxytocin. This was a new step in the pharmacological control of the birth process. First this synthetic hormone was available for intra-muscular injections. It became immediately popular during labour and for the delivery of the placenta, although the effects could not be easily controlled and the risks of fetal distress were high. Within a short time of the introduction of synthetic oxytocin, thanks to the replacement of gum pipes by plastic pipes, intravenous drips became much safer and appeared as the most effective and safest way to inject synthetic oxytocin.

The fashion of teaching women how to give birth

While these technical, scientific and pharmacological advances were strengthening the power of the obstetrician, an unprecedented and sophisticated form of culturally controlled childbirth suddenly appeared in the 1950s. It became fashionable to teach women how to give birth, and particularly how to breathe during labour and delivery. A disciple of Pavlov, the neuro-psychiatrist Velvovski, created in 1949 the 'psychoprophylactic method' to eliminate the pain of childbirth. The French obstetrician Lamaze introduced this method in Western countries. It became, in the USA, the 'Lamaze Method'. This method was based on the concepts of conditioned reflexes. The main theoretical basis was that the pain of labour is not physiological, but reflex-conditional and therefore cultural. The promoters of this method had understood that conditioned reflexes are related to the activity of the neocortex where all inhibitions come from in childbirth, but they had not understood that a reduction of the activity of the neocortex is the most important aspect of birth physiology among humans. They have not understood that a woman in labour must be protected against any sort of neocortical stimulation and that she must forget what she has learnt. Instead they thought that pregnant women have to be reconditioned through education and that labouring women need to be guided via the use of language.

Directly or indirectly, the influence of this method based on the work of theoreticians has been – and still is – enormous all over the world. Instead of identifying the basic needs of women in labour in order to facilitate the birth process and therefore to reduce the need for drugs and intervention, the focus was on the elimination of pain and fear via non-pharmacological 'methods'. The ambition of some obstetricians was to attach their name to such 'methods', in the same way that those of the previous generations had given their names to style of forceps. New actors entered the birth territory: 'monitrices d'accouchement sans douleur', helpers, guides, 'coaches', physiotherapists, psychologists. The conditioning of new generations of mothers was that women are not able to give birth without the guidance of an expert. The word 'privacy' was ignored. The reason for authentic midwifery was ignored. The socialization of childbirth had entered a new phase of its long history.

During the 1960s, technical, scientific, pharmacological and conceptual advances of the previous decade were gradually integrated into practice. The concentration of births in hospitals was an established fact. European midwives were remarkably silent. American midwives were almost completely forgotten. However the media and the general public became suddenly more interested in childbirth. French intellectuals, who had ignored observations by an experienced practitioner such as Grantly Dick Read, were fascinated by methods inspired by Pavlovian theoreticians. Mothers started to publish books inspired by their own experience. In the USA, Marjorie Karmel published her famous book 'Thank you, Dr Lamaze' in 1960, while in the UK, Sheila Kitzinger was writing 'The Experience of Childbirth'. There were open discussions among obstetricians about the new methods of preparation. Many of them were indifferent; some were ironic – 'just a fashion', while others

---

Box 9.4   Questions for discussion

- What do you think of the idea of teaching women how to have natural childbirth?
- What do you think about the cultural conditioning of childbirth?
- Do you believe there is a place for experts with birthing women? Why?

were enthusiastic. Meanwhile a new generation of surgically trained gynaecologists and obstetricians was emerging. Birth outcomes were evaluated through well-defined criteria, such as perinatal mortality rates, perinatal morbidity rates and maternal morbidity rates. Birth statistics were better and better. Obstetrics was not a second-class medical discipline any more. Obstetricians had established their territory.

THE ELECTRONIC AGE

The contemporary history of obstetrics is going so fast that every decade may be presented as a turning point and must be looked at separately. During the 1970s obstetrics entered the electronic age. Obstetricians enthusiastically rushed towards the first electronic fetal monitors available so that, within some years, these new machines were widely used all over the world. The dream of all obstetricians has always been to control the birth process in order to be ready to intervene as quickly as possible.

Electronic fetal monitoring appeared as a way to fulfil this widespread dream and as the key to the elimination of all risks in childbirth. Thanks to a printed graph, the obstetrician could control and discuss the decisions of other members of staff at any time of day and night. European midwives, like American obstetric nurses, became expert-technicians in the interpretation of data provided by the electronic monitor. Babies were born in a 'high-tech' environment.

Fathers invade the birth territory

Women had always given birth in mostly female environments. In the 1970s, within some years, the environment became more male than ever, not only because the number of (male) obstetricians was increasing, and not only because technology is a male symbol, but with the emergence of new doctrines. Within some years the doctrine was established that the baby's father must participate in the birth. Historically, the participation of the father cannot be dissociated from the concentration of births in 'high-tech' hospitals. Having men at birth appeared as a way for birthing women to adapt to absolutely new situations. The basis of the new theory was that the participation of the father, by creating strong ties inside the

Box 9.5   Questions for discussion

- What do you think about the role of men at birth?
- What effect of the partner's presence do you see on labouring women?

couple, would reduce the number of divorces and separations. It was also thought that the presence of a familiar person – such as the husband or the partner – would make the birth easier: the need for intervention should decrease. Many men were obviously reassured by the electronic surveillance of the birth process and the presence of an obstetrician. It did not take very long for the obstetrical milieus to assimilate the new doctrine. Meanwhile the number of babies alive and healthy at birth had increased, while the rates of caesareans and other interventions were climbing.

The masculinization of childbirth

There were of course geographical variations in the masculinisation of childbirth, which is a characteristic of that decade. The new tendencies were originally stronger in North America, where rates of caesareans were going up faster. In Ireland, on the other hand, fathers remained excluded from maternity units and rates of caesareans remained as low as 4% during the whole decade. In Holland, rates of home birth remained above 30%; birth statistics improved as quickly as in the neighbouring countries, without a significant increase in rates of intervention. In spite of such geographical variations, we can claim that at the end of the 1970s the territory of the obstetrician was vast, well-defined and apparently unchallenged – at least from the point of view of those whose horizon was limited to the conventional departments of obstetrics.

Environmental factors begin to be of concern – the call for a return to out–of–hospital birth

Interestingly, as soon as the electronic age began establishing itself, the importance of environmental factors during childbirth started to be recognized. In the USA, there was the beginning of a tendency towards out-of-hospital births. As early as 1971, in California, a number of women set up the Santa Cruz Birth Center. Soon after, in 1975, the creation of a free standing birthing centre by the 'Maternity Center Association' was approved by the New York State Department of Health. There was also a demand for home births. A new generation of lay midwives suddenly appeared, particularly in California. The hippies who left San Francisco and went 'out to save the world' eventually created the Farm, in Tennessee. Among them was Ina May Gaskin (Gaskin 1976).

At the same time, in France, in the context of the Pithiviers General Hospital, we were trying to 'bring the home inside the hospital' (Odent 1976; Gillett 1979). We transformed a conventional delivery room into a small home-like birthing room, in which there was no bed, no table, and no visible medical equipment – 'la salle sauvage'. In another room, we installed a paddling pool (the ancestor of hospital birthing pools), assuming that immersion in water at body temperature would reduce levels of adrenaline, and therefore reduce the need for drugs in the case of difficult labours. We also bought a piano, so that every Tuesday, pregnant women could meet and sing together, creating an opportunity to become familiar with the place and with members of the staff.

AFTER 1980 – THE EPIDURAL 'EVOLUTION'

While electronic fetal monitoring was introduced and became popular within some years, epidural anaesthesia became popular through a long 'evolution' rather than a 'revolution'. Even though the epidural technique had been known since the early 1900s, and although the first epidural catheters were inserted in the 1940s (Hingson 1944), the use of this method of regional analgesia in obstetrics had been sporadic until 1980. There had been several obstacles to its widespread use, even after the advent of plastic epidural catheters replacing ureteral catheters and of plastic intravenous catheters making safer the pre-block fluid loading. Until recently, only a very small number of anaesthesiologists were familiar with the obstetrical context and available day and night. Furthermore, many obstetricians resented another physician intruding with the parturient and therefore threatening their territory.

These obstacles were overcome around 1980. The widespread use of electronic fetal monitoring was associated with an increased use of oxytocin stimulation and an increased rate of caesareans. Obstetricians became less reluctant to involve anaesthetists, understanding the advantages of having an epidural catheter in place when deciding to do a caesarean. It was also a time when a new generation of physicians were being trained in obstetric anaesthesiology. All large hospitals could offer a continuous service, making possible the use of epidurals 24 hours a day. In addition, apart from countries such as Holland and Japan, there was an increased demand from mothers (and fathers). This is how obstetric anaesthesiology became a new medical discipline, with national and international societies and specialized journals. Newly trained doctors developed the many technical advances of the 1980s and 1990s. One advance was the association of a local anaesthetic and an opiate which led to the concept of 'walking epidurals'. Different ways to combine spinal and epidural anaesthesia could be adapted to a great variety of situations.

While the obstetric anaesthesiologist (more often than not, a man) was encroaching on the (spatial) territory of the obstetrician and interfering in the relationship with the parturient, others were eroding more insidiously the recently acquired high status of the obstetrician. Widespread use of electronic fetal monitoring had been based on a belief about its usefulness to diagnose fetal distress. Most obstetricians had shared the pre-conceived idea that continuously recording fetal heartbeats on a graph would improve statistics. They were just thinking of the advantages of a technique leading to an early diagnosis of fetal distress during labour. It is only when the electronic age was well-established that epidemiologists challenged pre-conceived ideas by publishing results of controlled studies comparing the effects of continuous monitoring versus intermittent auscultation on outcome statistics. In 1987, an authoritative review article of all these studies made clear that the only constant and significant effect on statistics of electronic fetal monitoring is to increase rates of caesareans, both in low-risk and in high-risk populations (Prentice and Lind 1987). In other words the ratio of benefits to risks is negative.

Most practitioners could not anticipate such results. They were not in a position to understand that the only fact that a woman in labour knows is that her body functions are continuously monitored, which tends to stimulate her neocortex and therefore to make the birth longer, more difficult and therefore more dangerous, so that finally more babies need to be rescued by more caesareans. With such studies we were entering the age of evidence-based obstetrics.

TODAY – PRENATALLY

Today the number of actors involved in childbirth is rapidly increasing, and the limits of the territory of each of them are imprecise and unsettled. It is as if every actor is gradually eroding the territory and the autonomy of the obstetrician. The situation is still more confused, because the territory of the obstetrician was traditionally male, while the territory of the midwife was traditionally female. Nowadays, there are many female obstetricians and even some male midwives.

After introducing the concept of medicalized antenatal care during the twentieth century, obstetricians had significantly enlarged their territory. General practitioners and midwives who remained involved in prenatal surveillance were in fact practising as the proxy of the obstetricians. Obstetricians had designed exemplary batteries of routine exams and routine tests which general practitioners and midwives had to carry out. With the advent of ultrasound imaging and the development of multiple screening and diagnostic tests, the central role of the obstetrician in antenatal care became apparently irreplaceable and therefore unchallenged.

Obstetric territory is now under siege

At the dawn of the twenty-first century, this huge annexed territory of the obstetrician is suddenly threatened. To begin with, there are reasons for reconsidering the very concept of routine medicalized antenatal care. Also there is a risk of fragmentation related to the emergence of new medical disciplines. Traditional patterns of medical care were based on the belief that more antenatal visits mean better outcomes. They were not based on scientific data. Today, hard evidence leads us to reconsider these pre-conceived ideas.

British studies failed to find any association between late enrollment in prenatal care (after 28 weeks gestation) and either adverse maternal or neonatal outcomes (Thomas et al 1991) or between the number of visits and the onset of eclampsia (Douglas and Redmond 1994). These studies cast doubts on the efficacy of such protocols. Within the British National Health Service, the number of visits is not as strongly associated with socio-economic status as it is in the USA. This makes the results of the British studies comparatively easier to interpret than those of the American studies (Vintzileos et al 2002a,b). However, it is worth analysing the Center for Disease Control and Prevention (CDC) in the USA's Morbidity and Mortality Weekly report dated 6 December 2002. This report indicates that women who were born outside the USA are more likely than their racial and ethnic counterparts born in the USA to begin prenatal care late or to have no prenatal care at all. 'In spite of that' (or perhaps 'because of that'?) women born in the United States are more likely than their counterparts born outside the United States to give birth preterm (11.9% versus 10.5%) or to give birth to a low weight baby (7.9% versus 6.4%).

It is also fruitful to analyse trials comparing different schedules of antenatal visits. One was conducted in California, in a Kaiser Permanente Medical Center (Binstock et al 1995). A second trial, in South East London, involved 2794 women (Sikorski et al 1996). A third one, by WHO, involved 53 centres in Thailand, Cuba, Saudi Arabia and Argentina (Villar et al 2001). None of these trials demonstrated any benefits of conventional schedules compared with reduced visit schedules.

One may also wonder if women who have a great number of antenatal visits give birth more easily than those with none. For obvious reasons, a randomized trial is impossible. A study on the effect of cocaine use on the progress of labour unexpectedly suggested the opposite (Wehbeh et al 1995). The researchers took into account that one-third of cocaine users had no prenatal care, versus 4% of non-users. It was therefore essential to determine the average dilation at admission among non-users of cocaine who had no prenatal care. It appeared that the mean dilation at admission in this group was

Box 9.6   Questions for discussion

• What do you make of the fact that women who didn't have any antenatal care were more likely to be further dilated on admission than those who did have antenatal care?

5.4 cm, whereas it was 3.8 cm among those who had more than four antenatal visits (it was 4.63 cm for cocaine users).

The content of antenatal visits must also be reconsidered. Not long ago, the main reason for the first antenatal visit was to establish the diagnosis of pregnancy. Today, in the age of reliable pregnancy tests that are bought over-the-counter, this primary reason for an early antenatal visit has disappeared. Routine ultrasound scanning, the symbol of modern prenatal care and its most expensive component, has been reconsidered after the results of studies comparing the effects on birth outcomes of routine ultrasound screening versus the selective use of scans. One of these randomized trials, published in the New England Journal of Medicine, led to an unequivocal conclusion: 'The findings of this study clearly indicate that ultrasound screening does not improve perinatal outcome in current US practice' (Ewigman et al 1993). Authors of a meta-analysis came to similar conclusions: 'Routine ultrasound scanning does not improve the outcome of pregnancy in terms of an increased number of live births or of reduced perinatal morbidity. Routine ultrasound scanning may be effective and useful as a screening for malformation. Its use for this purpose, however, should be made explicit and take into account the risk of false positive diagnosis in addition to ethical issues' (Bucher and Schmidt 1993). One of the effects of a selective use of ultrasounds is to dramatically reduce the number of scans, particularly in the vulnerable phase of early pregnancy. Even in a high-risk population of pregnant women, ultrasound scans are not as useful as commonly believed. Evidence from randomised controlled trials suggests that sonographic identification of fetal growth restriction does not improve outcome despite increased medical surveillance (Secher et al 1987; Larson and Larson 1992). In diabetic pregnancies it has been demonstrated that ultrasound measurements are not more accurate than clinical examination in identifying high birth weight babies (Johnstone et al 1996). This led to the memorable title of an editorial in the British Journal of Obstetrics and Gynaecology: 'Guess the weight of the baby' (1996).

At the same time, a huge Canadian study demonstrated that the only effect of routine glucose tolerance screening was to inform 2.7% of pregnant women that they have gestational diabetes (Wen et al 2000). The diagnosis did not change birth outcomes. Even the efficacy of haemoglobin concentration to detect anaemia and iron deficiency is being reconsidered because haemoglobin concentration indicates the degree of blood dilution, an effect of placental activity.

Reconsidering both the concept of routine medicalized antenatal care, and the content of antenatal visits, leads us to re-examine the reason for antenatal care. From the point of view of most expectant mothers the primary question should be: 'What can the obstetrician do for me and my baby, since I already know I am pregnant, I don't have any chronic health condition, and I can feel the baby growing?' The simplified answer is: 'Not a lot, apart from detecting a gross abnormality and offering an abortion'. At a time when we might expect a decline of medicalized care in pregnancy, we can also expect a rise of *preconceptional counselling*, including nutritional advice (Odent 2002). We should not conclude that there is no need at all for medical examinations in pregnancy: we cannot make a comprehensive list of all the reasons why women might need the advice or the help of a qualified health professional before giving birth. It is the word 'routine' that should be discarded in the current scientific context.

Box 9.7   Questions for discussion

• What do you think are the implications of these contentions about the 'routine' aspect of antenatal care?
• What are the responsibilities of healthcare practitioners and governments in providing health services for childbearing women?

A new territory emerges – maternal fetal medicine

It is important to think about women who want to detect possible fetal abnormalities. This leads us to consider the increased number and current territory of fetal medicine specialists. They practice in large hospitals. They have expertise and sophisticated equipment available to provide valuable answers. They work in cooperation with specialists in genetic counseling, whose domain is quite precise and expanding. The limits of the territory of fetal medicine specialists, on the other hand, are highly dependent on technological advances. For example, it appears today that fetal trophoblasts can be recovered from cervical secretions, so that prenatal diagnosis could be done via a simple Pap smear at 6 weeks. At least three teams of researchers (in Brisbane, Paris, and Israel) are well advanced in exploring this approach. When such a definitive and non-invasive test is available, the daily life of fetal medicine specialists will be radically different.

We must also think of pregnant women with a pre-existing medical condition. This leads us to consider the emerging field of obstetric medicine on both sides of the Atlantic. While the North American Society of Obstetric Medicine was created, handbooks of obstetric medicine were published in Europe (Nelson-Piercy 2001). One of the reasons for this new discipline is that today women with conditions such as cystic fibrosis, insulin-dependent diabetes, or congenital heart disease can reach adulthood and become pregnant. Others have pre-existing chronic medical conditions including, in particular, rheumatic disorders and severe, chronic hypertension. Some pregnant women are survivors of life-threatening diseases, such as cancers and leukemia. It has been claimed recently that every woman with cancer should be offered the chance to preserve her fertility by 'banking' an ovary. There are pregnant women who have had an organ transplant and are treated by immunosuppressants. The role of obstetric medicine now extends to medical problems in pregnancy such as cholestasis and thromboembolism. The emergence and fast development of obstetric medicine is to a great extent related to delayed childbirth and reduced fertility. There are strong links between internists practising obstetric medicine and fertility specialists. The population of pregnant women is getting older and sicker. We must realize that the effectiveness of our modern medical treatments, including assisted reproduction technologies, is reversing the laws of natural selection. We must start looking at the magnificent medical miracles of our time from a long-term public health perspective.

Obstetrician as a primary caregiver

The current evolution of antenatal care explains that in many countries the obstetrician is now considered a primary caregiver. But even this role is challenged, particularly in countries, such as Germany, where more and more independent midwives reclaim an increased autonomy. In the age of medicalized antenatal care, there is an unexpected reason for a revival of the historical rivalry between midwives and obstetricians.

TODAY – PERINATALLY

In the perinatal period, there are enormous differences in the roles of obstetricians, (according to the country), to the ratio of midwives to obstetricians, to whether the practice is urban or rural, to the standard of living of the population, to the size of the maternity unit, to the concomitant practice of gynaecology, and to the mode of practice (public or private). In terms of spatial territory, it is difficult to compare countries where the caesarean is a common way to give birth (such as China, India, Brazil, Mexico, and other Latin American countries), and countries (such as Holland, Russia, and Japan) where the vaginal route is still by far the most common way.

Since, at a global level, rates of caesareans are high, and since many obstetricians also practice gynaecologic surgery, we might be tempted to claim that today, the obstetrician is at home in the operating theatre. In fact the modern operating theatre is a territory the obstetrician must share with other physicians, particularly the obstetric anaesthesiologist and the neonatologist. When neonatology separated from general paediatrics, obstetricians and midwives were still in charge of neonatal emergencies, particularly occasional resuscitations. The first rare specialists in this new discipline were receiving babies transferred to their units. Today neonatologists are more and more visible in operating theatres. Some of them even consider themselves perinatologists. We might make similar comments about the modern delivery room, where the obstetric anaesthesiologist is often more visible than the obstetrician, and where the neonatologist is welcome.

The invisible threat to the autonomy and authority of the obstetrician

In reality, these visible actors in the delivery room and the operating theatre do not seriously threaten the autonomy of the obstetrician. The threat comes mostly from invisible actors. Modern obstetricians must submit to implied rules established by lawyers, judges, and insurance companies. They are more or less, prisoners of guidelines, protocols, and recommendations established by committees. Such committees are influenced by the dogma of evidence-based medicine, which is mainly promoted by public-health researchers and epidemiologists. Evidence-based medicine is a precious tool at the service of practitioners. As a dogma, it becomes counterproductive, disregarding the value of experience and skill, and pushing out creative, inquiring and innovative minds.

At the same time, we must not underestimate the power of the media and the influence of consumer groups as promoters of concepts of choice in childbirth and of birth plans. On the same day, an obstetrician may have to adapt to demands as diverse as 'I want to give birth with nobody else around than my doula', or 'I want to schedule a caesarean birth'. An accumulation of factors tends to 'instrumentalize' the obstetrician. Meanwhile, in the USA in particular, the recruitment of young obstetricians has decreased steadily since the beginning of the twenty first century. The slight decline of the US birthrates cannot provide a relevant explanation.

THE FUTURE

The way babies will be born during the next decades – and therefore the role of the obstetrician – will depend to a great extent on the criteria used to evaluate obstetric and midwifery practices.

First scenario

One of the most plausible scenarios in the near future is that the battery of conventional criteria will remain unchanged. This means that public health organizations, practitioners, and all those involved in childbirth will have to take into account the results of studies that ignore criteria other than perinatal mortality and morbidity rates, maternal morbidity rates and cost effectiveness. If such a scenario prevails, we can anticipate that in the near future the caesarean section will become the most common way to give birth, even the norm. This is already true for a great part of humanity. We must keep in mind recent technical advances that make the operation more simple, faster, and safer (Odent 2004). Let us recall that in the 1990s Michael Stark and the team of the Misgav Ladach Hospital in Jerusalem, developed a method of caesarean section that restricts the use of sharp instruments, preferring manual manipulation instead, and removes every unnecessary step, such as suturing the peritoneum. The advantages in terms of speed, blood loss, and therefore safety are indisputable. We must also constantly keep in mind the current widespread and quasi cultural lack of understanding of birth physiology, and therefore of the basic needs of labouring women.

In such a context we may expect more and more studies demonstrating that, whatever the situation, a caesarean birth is always the safest approach in well-equipped obstetrical units, according to conventional criteria. Such studies may involve self-selected groups, for example, women who had an elective caesarean on demand; they may also be prospective and randomized, inspired by the famous multicentre trial about breech presentation at term.

Wherever caesarean section is the most common way to give birth, the obstetricians are mostly surgeons, and also primary care givers for pregnant women. Their territory is double: office and operating theatre.

Differences will remain between countries regarding who attends the birth of women who want to try the vaginal route. In countries where midwifery is not well-established, it seems that the emergence of a new actor is imminent. Ten hospital systems in the United States have already started or are about to start using so-called 'laborists', according to a report at the 2005 annual meeting of the American College of Obstetricians and Gynecologists. Laborists are physicians in charge of 'labour management'. This implies that all labours are supposed to be 'managed'. They work in shifts. The 'laborist' profession can offer private obstetricians and gynaecologists less disruption to their office and operating room schedules. We don't need to invent the future. It is already here.

Second scenario

The deep-rooted intuitive knowledge still shared by some women (and even some men) will lead them to perceive the limits of our conventional ways to evaluate how babies are born.

Transmission of this intuitive knowledge will be facilitated by the powerful support provided by recent scientific advances. It will appear that we need to learn to think long-term and to think in terms of civilization where childbirth is concerned. In other words, we'll perceive scientifically-based reasons to enlarge our batteries of criteria when evaluating midwifery and obstetric practices.

Our 'Primal Health Research Data Bank' may be presented as a tool in order to train ourselves to think long-term (www.birthworks.org/primalhealth). Primal Health Research is a developing branch of epidemiology that explores correlations between what happens at the beginning of our life and what will happen later on in terms of health and behaviour (the beginning of our life is defined as the 'primal period', which includes fetal life, the perinatal period and the year following birth) (Odent 1986). From an overview of this database, we can differentiate the important subgroup of studies detecting risk factors in the perinatal period for health conditions and behaviours that express themselves in childhood, adolescence and adulthood. It is noticeable that when researchers explore a disease or a way of being that can be interpreted as an 'impaired capacity to love', they always detect risk factors in the perinatal period. 'Impaired capacity to love' is a convenient term to establish links between these studies, because it can include the capacity to love others and the capacity to love oneself as well; it can include self-destructive behaviours. It explains why we classify 'Primal Health Research' among the scientific disciplines that participate in 'The Scientification of Love'. Among key words leading to such studies, let us mention juvenile criminality, suicide, drug addiction, anorexia nervosa, autism…many highly topical issues.

'The Scientification of Love' leads us to think not only long-term, but also in terms of civilization (Odent 1999). Until recently, love was a topic for poets, novelists, philosophers and lay people. Today it is studied from multiple scientific perspectives. Disciplines that participate in this vital aspect of the current scientific revolution, include, apart from Primal Health Research, ethology, animal experiments, the study of the behavioural effects of hormones involved in all the different facets of love, and also inter-cultural comparisons. The scientification of love provides answers to paradoxically new questions such as: 'How does the capacity to love develop?' Today, a combination of data converges to give great importance to early experiences, particularly in the period surrounding birth. We are learning that the short phase of labour between the birth of the baby and delivery of the placenta is probably critical in the development of the capacity to love.

Interestingly, it is this 'third stage of labour' that is the most commonly disturbed by all cultural milieus, via a great diversity of beliefs and rituals. The most universal and intriguing way to disturb the first contact between mother and baby is simply to promote the belief that colostrum is tainted or harmful to the baby. Several beliefs and rituals can be combined and can reinforce each other. The cost of such beliefs and rituals is enormous in terms of post-partum haemorrhage and maternal death. These practices hinder the release of the vital high peak of oxytocin mothers have the capacity to reach, if the first contact between mother and baby is not disturbed. However these disrupting rituals and beliefs probably have evolutionary advantages since they are quasi-universal.

One must keep in mind that for thousands of years, the basic strategy for survival of most human groups has been to dominate nature and to dominate other human groups. There was an evolutionary advantage in developing the human potential for aggression rather than the capacity to love and therefore in transmitting such beliefs and rituals. It is significant, when comparing different societies, that the greater the need to develop aggression and the ability to destroy life, the more intrusive the rituals and cultural beliefs are in the neonatal period.

Our interpretations must be framed in the context of the twenty-first century. We are at a time when Humanity must invent radical new strategies for survival. Today we are in the process of realizing the limits of traditional strategies. We must raise new questions such as: 'how to develop this form of love which is respect for Mother Earth?' In order to stop destroying the planet we need a sort of unification of the planetary village. We need love more than ever before. All these beliefs and rituals are suddenly losing their evolutionary advantages. In the age of the 'Scientification of Love', there are new reasons to improve our understanding of the physiological processes, in order to disturb them as little as possible. There are serious reasons to introduce new criteria in order to evaluate how babies are born.

Only if – rediscovering the basic needs of birthing women and newborn babies

The introduction of such new criteria will have practical implications, only if the basic needs of birthing women and newborn babies are rediscovered. This will be the difficult point after thousands of years of culturally controlled childbirth. A better understanding of the physiological processes will go hand in hand with the emergence of authentic midwifery. The midwife will be understood as a mother figure whose first responsibility is to protect the privacy of the mother-to-be. When authentic midwifery is rediscovered, obstetricians can recover their genuine role as experts in unusual and pathological situations. There is no reason for rivalries between authentic midwives and authentic obstetricians. The limits of their respective territories are well defined.

Then the history of childbirth will enter a new phase. Until now it has been the history of rivalries inside cultural milieus to control physiological processes.

Summary Box

- The territory of the obstetrician is eminently unstable and imprecise. This is why physiological, historical, and geographical perspectives must be combined before analysing the current global situation and before looking towards the future.
- After a long history of rivalry between the midwife and the medical man, the autonomy of the obstetrician is suddenly threatened by the emergence of a great diversity of new actors in the field of pregnancy and childbirth (development of obstetric anaesthesiology, neonatology, perinatology, fetal medicine, obstetric medicine, genetic counselling, epidemiology and 'evidence-based obstetrics', public health, alternative medicine), concomitant with the increased power of the media, the consumer groups, the judges and lawyers, and the insurance companies...
- The future of obstetrics depends on its capacity to introduce new criteria to evaluate how human beings are born. 'Primal Health Research' leads to the introduction of long-term criteria. 'The Scientification of Love' leads society to think in terms of civilization.

References

Binstock MA, Wolde-Tsadik G 1995 Alternative prenatal care: impact of reduced visit frequency, focused visits and continuity of care. Journal of Reproductive Medicine 40: 507–512.

Bordahl PE, Hem E 1998 An appropriate forceps – 150-year anniversary of Simpson's forceps. Tidsskr Nor Laegeforen 118(30): 4662–4665. [Article in Norwegian].

Bucher HC, Schmidt JG 1993 Does routine ultrasound scanning improve outcome in pregnancy? Meta-analysis of various outcome measures. British Medical Journal 307: 13–17.

Donnison J 1977 Midwives and Medical Men, Heinemann, London.

Douglas KA & Redman CW 1994 Eclampsia in the United Kingdom. British Medical Journal, 309:1395–1400.

Eaton SB, Shostak M, Konner M 1988 The Paleolithic prescription. Harper and Row, New York.

Edmunds J 1866 Inaugural Address. Lancet 1:613–614.

Ewigman BG, Crane JP, Frigoletto FD et al 1993 Effect of prenatal ultrasound screening on perinatal outcome. New England Journal of Medicine, 329:821–827.

Gaskin IM 1976 Spiritual midwifery.

Gillett J 1979 Childbirth in Pithiviers, France. Lancet 2: 894–896.

Hingson RA, Southword JL 1944 Continuous peridural anesthesia. Anesthesia Analgesia 23(5): 215–227.

Johnstone FD, Prescott RJ, Steel JM et al 1996 Clinical and ultrasound prediction of macrosomia in diabetic pregnancy. British Journal of Obstetrics and Gynaecology 103: 747–754.

Kerr JMM 1926 The technique of cesarean section, with special reference to the lower uterine segment incision. American Journal of Obstetrics and Gynecology 12: 729–734.

Larson T, Larson FJ 1992 Detection of small-for-gestational-age fetuses by ultrasound screening in a high risk population: a randomized controlled study, British Journal of Obstetrics and Gynaecology 99: 469–474.

Nelson-Piercy C 2001Handbook of obstetric medicine. Taylor & Francis, London.

Nissen E, Lilja G, Widstrom AM, Uvnas-Moberg K 1995 Elevation of oxytocic levels early postpartum in women. Acta Obstetrica Gynecologica Scandanavia 74: 530–533.

Odent M 1976 Bien naître. Le Seuil, Paris.

Odent M 1986 Primal health. Century-Hutchinson, London.

Odent M 1987 The fetus ejection reflex. Birth 14: 104–105.

Odent M 1999 The Scientification of Love, Free Association Books, London.

Odent M 2002 The rise of preconceptional counselling vs the decline of medicalized care in pregnancy. Primal Health Research Newsletter 10(3): 1–6.

Odent M 2004 The caesarean. Free Association Books, London.

Prentice A, Lind T 1987 Fetal heart monitoring during labour – too frequent intervention, too little benefit. Lancet 2: 1375–1377.

Secher NJ, Kern Hansen P 1987 A randomized study of fetal abdominal diameter and fetal weight estimation for detection of light-for-gestation infants in low-risk pregnancy. British Journal of Obstetrics and Gynaecology 94: 105.

Schiefenhovel W 1978 Childbirth among the Eipos, New Guinea. Film presented at the Congress of Ethnomedicine, Gottingen, Germany.

Sikorski J, Wilson J, Clement S et al 1996 A randomised controlled trial comparing two schedules of antenatal visits: The antenatal project. British Medical Journal 312: 546–553.

Thomas P, Golding J, Peters TJ 1991 Delayed antenatal care: Does it affect pregnancy outcome? Social Science and Medicine, 32: 715–723.

Villar J, Ba'aqueel H, Piaggio G et al 2001 WHO antenatal care randomized trial for the evaluation of a new model of routine antenatal care. Lancet 357: 1551–1564.

Vintzileos AM, Ananth CV, Smulian JC et al 2002a The impact of prenatal care in the United States on preterm births in the presence or absence of antenatal high-risk conditions, American Journal of Obstetrics and Gynecology 187: 1254–1257.

Vintzileos AM, Ananth CV, Smulian JC et al 2002b The impact of prenatal care on postneonatal deaths in the presence or absence of antenatal high-risk conditions, American Journal of Obstetrics and Gynecology 187: 1258–1262.

Von Siebold ECJ 1839 Versuch einer Geschichte der Gerburtshulfe, Berlin.

Wehbeh H, Matthews RP, McCalla S et al 1995 The effect of recent cocaine use on the progress of labor. American Journal of Obstetrics and Gynecology 172: 1014–1018.

Wen SW, Liu S, Kramer MS et al 2000 Impact of prenatal glucose screening on the diagnosis of gestational diabetes and on pregnancy outcomes. American Journal of Epidemiology 152(11): 1009–1014.

Wood P, Foureur M 2005 Exploring the maternity archive of the St Helens Hospital, Wellington, New Zealand, 1907–22: An historian and a midwife collaborate. In: B Mortimer, S McGann (Eds). New directions in the history of nursing: International perspectives. Routledge Studies in the Social History of Medicine, London.

Chapter **10**

From ideal to real: The interface between birth territory and the maternity service organization

Pat Brodie
Nicky Leap

INTRODUCTION

This chapter will explore issues associated with the notions of 'birth territory and midwifery guardianship' in relation to the every day reality of working within maternity services. Using examples from our experience of improving the quality of birthing territory for women and midwives in Australia and the United Kingdom, we will explore philosophical, organizational and cultural change strategies that we consider are necessary for the successful implementation of woman-centred birth territory within publicly funded maternity services in Western countries. (These strategies will be highlighted in text boxes throughout the chapter.) We will also examine the role of leadership in making these changes happen and the value of collaborative relationships in enabling optimum experiences for women and their families.

Processes involving change often start with developing an understanding of what would be 'ideal' and then planning for what is possible within limited, existing budgets. It is often outside of the realms of possibility to carry out a major makeover of the birthing area in a maternity unit in order to promote privacy and physiological processes for labouring women. In this chapter, we will explore some low budget, practical options that can be implemented in any setting. However, creating 'the right environment' for birthing is about far more than the material objects that are installed (or removed) with good intentions. In order for women to benefit from such initiatives, we believe that it is necessary for midwives to have a clear understanding of what would be ideal birthing territory, in terms of their guardianship role in the promotion of physiology and woman-centred approaches to practice.

Bridging the gap between idealism and 'the real world' requires strategies to change the culture in maternity services that are a mixture of practical and philosophical considerations, grounded in practice, but nevertheless, aimed at stimulating the imagination of all involved in providing services, raising possibilities and promoting action. The most obvious strategy is to remove the majority of services away from institutions and into the community.

We will explore the importance of promoting community based services, home birth and birth centres later in this chapter. However, it is essential that we look at ways of changing the culture in the environment where the majority of women give birth – the places usually referred to as 'labour wards' and 'delivery suites' – if we are to make any impact on the majority of women's lives. This will involve a multi-faceted approach, one that involves changing the environment in which midwifery is enacted, the nature of practice, the systems of care and the relationships of key players. Support of such changes needs to be articulated at every level, particularly in policy documents and routes of funding.

In our experience, it is only when midwives are able to critique the barriers to the 'ideal' and understand the power dynamics of the contexts in which they practise, that they are able to come together with others to strategize around changing systems and cultures. This requires a political approach to practice, the importance of which has been identified by Eugene Declercq:

> 'Midwives' roles were diminished over the last century not because of their failure as caregivers but because of their failure to respond to the political challenges they faced.' (Declercq 1994, p. 237)

It is essential that midwives are able to identify the value of midwifery in places where policy decisions are made. In our experience, one of the key factors in being able to introduce any changes in maternity service provision has been being able to show that such initiatives were part of the new directions that government policies were recommending. This is why it is important that all midwifery education programs address the politics of midwifery and the knowledge and skills midwives need to function as change agents in promoting woman-centred services. Furthermore, enabling such a profound shift in the culture and organization of maternity services requires strong midwifery leadership.

THE LANGUAGE OF 'NORMAL' BIRTH

An examination of the language and concepts that are used in relation to birth territory and midwifery guardianship will set the scene for our practical suggestions for reform in maternity service provision. We argue that promoting understanding of how language and philosophical concepts are translated into actions is the first step in making changes happen that benefit childbearing women.

Raising awareness about language is not just about promoting the use of words that are respectful and effective communication tools; the language we use both reflects and constructs the culture in which we practise (Bastian 1992; Leap 1992; Hewison 1993; Hastie 2005). Questioning the potential subconscious effects of the language we use is important. For example, Holly Powell Kennedy (2004) has suggested that the

---

Box 10.1 Changing the culture of maternity services

- Understanding issues of power and control and how this affects birth.
- Conceptualizing the 'ideal' and a philosophy of woman centred midwifery before planning for possibilities.
- Stimulating the imagination of all involved in providing services in order to promote action.
- Recognizing the value of midwifery and 'community' when changing systems.
- Addressing forces that constrain midwifery and collaborative relationships.
- The imperative for midwives to be political and influence policy and for strong midwifery leadership.

notion of 'normal' is hardly in keeping with the midwifery philosophy of embracing the concept of each woman's birth being viewed by her as essentially 'special'. In this chapter, the phrases 'promoting physiological birth' and 'promoting a social model of birth' are deliberately used as well as variations of the commonly heard phrase: 'the midwifery art of keeping birth normal'. However, we are mindful that women and most maternity care providers are unlikely to use the terms 'physiological' and 'social'. The word 'normal' is embedded in the documentation and discourses that shape and reflect contemporary maternity service provision. Importantly, the term 'normal' is used to identify the primary domain of the midwife, a sphere of practice that is clearly defined as separate from the technological or medical interventions associated with complications, identified here by the World Health Organization (WHO):

> 'The midwife appears to be the most appropriate and cost effective type of care provider to be assigned to the care of normal pregnancy and birth, including risk assessment and the recognition of complications.' (World Health Organization 1996 p. 6)

In many Western countries the phrase, 'midwives are guardians of the normal' is used to summarize the role midwives play in the fraught arena of contemporary maternity service politics. The word 'guardian' suggests protection. For some, the phrase will be directly linked to the midwife's role in promoting a social model of birth and minimizing unnecessary contact with what has been called the 'technocratic' model of childbirth (Davis-Floyd 1994, 2001; Kitzinger 2000). For others, subconscious, religious images of guardian angels keeping at bay sinister forces may be triggered by the words, 'guardians of the normal'. However, we wish to acknowledge that it is not only doctors who hinder the promotion of physiology in technocratic systems. A polarized view that sees midwives as guardians who have to protect women from doctors is simplistic and does not allow all players to examine the role they play in promoting or hindering processes that can have a profound effect on women, their families and communities.

The process of raising awareness around language needs to be embedded in the education and practice of all those involved in maternity service provision. This can include light hearted innovations such as a fund raising jar in the workplace where practitioners contribute coins whenever they use words such as 'confinement' or 'delivery'. When engaging in multidisciplinary emergency drills, a fun approach that we have used is to personalize the mannequin and treat 'Monica' with respect. This provides an ideal situation in which to model and discuss communication that is woman-centred in a non-threatening way.

ENABLING 'WOMAN–CENTRED' BIRTH TERRITORY

In the last few decades, midwives have been addressing the complexity of their role in being 'with woman' and creating environments that promote physiological birth. This is often explained in terms of the potentially self-transformative nature of birth and the profound long-term consequences of empowerment for women, their families and society (Leap 2004; Leap and Anderson 2004). The promotion of woman-centred birth territory begins in early pregnancy and is about much more than aiming for an uncomplicated birth. It is concerned with a journey to motherhood that will have far-reaching consequences for each individual woman in terms of how she feels about herself, her body and her capabilities (Thompson 2004). Whether

---

Box 10.2   Raising consciousness about language

- Language describes and perpetuates technocratic systems.
- Language can promote 'woman-centred' approaches.
- Language can disempower and trivialize women and their experiences.
- Questioning the effect of the word 'normal' for women.
- The contribution of language to changing the culture of maternity services.
- Identifying opportunities in the workplace for raising consciousness about language and woman-centred care.

she eventually gives birth without intervention or not, a woman who feels powerful is in a good situation to take on becoming a new mother:

> 'Birth is not only about making babies. Birth is also about making mothers – strong, competent, capable mothers who trust themselves and know their inner strength.' (Katz-Rothman 1996, pp. 253–254)

Sadly the opposite is also true and women can end up feeling disempowered and emotionally fragile as a result of an experience of childbirth that rendered them passive in the face of interventionist approaches from a range of care providers (Kitzinger 2000). In order to minimize this happening, all practitioners need to have an understanding of what it means to put women at the centre of care.

'Woman-centred' midwifery is a concept that has been articulated by both the Royal College of Midwives in the United Kingdom (RCM 2001) and the Australian College of Midwives (ACM 2002). The concept has been used as the central tenet of the *ACM Philosophy Statement* (ACM 2004) and the Australian Nursing and Midwifery Council's *National Competency Standards for the Midwife* (ANMC 2006). Underpinning the concept of woman-centred midwifery is the community development notion that if you concentrate on enabling situations in which individual women can feel stronger, they, in turn, will enable situations in which their families and communities can feel more powerful. Understanding this is important when addressing common challenges to the notion such as, 'What about fathers/the baby/the woman's family?' Woman-centred midwifery is directly linked to feminist notions of empowerment and the transformative potential of birthing for women (Leap 2004). As such it is central to discussions about the impact of birth territory on women's experiences and lives. (It is interesting to note that comparable documents in the USA have chosen 'family-centred' rather than 'woman-centred' as a core tenet of practice. In Australia, many would feel more comfortable with 'family-centred' as inclusive nomenclature. The rationale for explaining 'woman-centred' as a concept is therefore often challenged in debates with health practitioners and academic colleagues.)

In the New Zealand setting – a society founded on the notion of 'partnership' – the focus of midwifery practice is more likely to be articulated as 'the partnership model'. This has been fully explained by midwifery leaders Karen Guilliland and Sally Pairman (1995) in their ground-breaking monograph *The midwifery partnership: A model for practice*. Whether the preferred nomenclature is 'partnership' or 'woman-centred care', there is an assumed feminist ethic underpinning the concept of placing the midwifery relationship with the woman at the centre of practice, as well as an explicit understanding of power sharing (Page 1993; Pairman 2000). We suggest that how these principles are enacted in practice raises questions that relate directly to birth territory and midwifery guardianship. In order to make these links, it is important to return to basic understandings regarding the nature of midwifery and the midwife-woman relationship (Kirkham 2000).

THE NATURE OF MIDWIFERY

> 'It is only with careful and systematic inquiry about the nature of midwifery care that the profession can clearly define and explicate a model of excellence that can be upheld as a standard for all women.' (Powell Kennedy et al 2004, p. 4)

The philosophy and particular nature of midwifery has been explored with practical references to an approach that:

- minimizes disturbance, direction, authority and intervention;
- maximizes the potential for physiology, common sense and instinctive behaviour to prevail;
- places trust in the expertise of the childbearing woman;
- shifts power towards the woman (Leap 2000, p. 2).

An exploration of this 'with woman' relationship includes a challenge to midwives to find ways to embrace uncertainty with women, to communicate that we believe in their expertise, and to avoid creating dependencies. Faye Thompson (2004) asserts that the promotion of self-determination through power sharing is directly related to the effective establishment of the mother-baby relationship. She describes the 'ethical journey' that is central to the woman–midwife relationship:

> 'The metaphor of journey… concerns the process of discovery and uncertainty and the impact of experiences associated with that journeying.' (Thompson 2004, p. 5)

The metaphor of a journey was also used by one of us (NL) in an attempt to explore the midwifery concept of 'the less we do, the more we give' (Leap 2000). This concept has been described by Holly Powell Kennedy (2000, p.12) as 'the art of doing "nothing" well'. Kennedy and colleagues engaged in a rigorous research process to illicit the qualities of what it is that is unique about exemplary midwifery (Powell Kennedy 2000, 2004; Powell Kennedy, Rousseau and Kane Low 2003; Powell Kennedy et al 2004). Three themes emerged from this research:

1. The midwife in relationship with the woman.
2. Orchestration of an environment of care.
3. The outcomes of care, called 'life journeys' for the woman and midwife.

Similar themes emerged when Kennedy and colleagues (2003) conducted a metasynthesis of six qualitative studies of midwifery practice in the USA. These findings offer a benchmark and structure for considering the midwifery relationship with women and behaviours that focus on the nature of 'being with' women and 'orchestrating' an appropriate environment rather than a set of 'doing to' tasks (Fahy 1998). These concepts can translate for an individual woman into the difference between a feeling that she 'gave birth', compared to a sense that she 'had it done to her'.

There is no doubt that women will never forget the role their midwife played as they engaged in this 'rite of passage', particularly the kind and unkind things that were said and done (Leap and Hunter 1993; Simkin 1999). It is not surprising therefore, that the concept of the midwife as 'guardian' – the person entrusted with ensuring emotional, physical and social safety for the woman – emerges as a concept in many cultures.

Understanding the nature of midwifery in terms of these philosophical underpinnings is an important first step in midwifery practice development initiatives. However, in order for midwives to practise according to these principles, the next step is to examine the 'real life' culture in which midwifery is practised. Recognition of the 'reality' midwives face in their day-to-day life in terms of issues pertaining to power and control is important if this is to happen.

IDEAL TO REAL: CHANGING THE CULTURE IN WHICH MIDWIFERY IS PRACTISED

We do not underestimate the difficulties of making change happen in a 'fragmented, hierarchical' system 'borrowed from the army and adapted for nursing' (Flint 1988; 1993, p. 25), a culture of medical dominance, horizontal violence, and oppressive power imbalances that stifle woman-centred care. Furthermore, since the majority of midwives are working in institutions with escalating caesarean section rates and where 'normal' birth is not necessarily the most common experience for women, it is imperative that we explore the tension between how we define our role and how it is played out in institutions if we are to institute major reforms in the way in which maternity services are organized.

An important study of 1464 births in five Consultant units in the United Kingdom (Downe, McCormick and Beech 2001) offers a snapshot of the grim realities of mainstream maternity service provision. After women who had artificial rupture of membranes; induction; acceleration; epidural anaesthesia; or episiotomy were

---

Box 10.3 Building respect and philosophical understandings about birth

- The potential for transformation: women, families, communities.
- Birth as a 'life journey' with profound consequences for all involved.
- Birth as a rite of passage.
- A social model of midwifery.
- The midwife's guardianship role.
- The woman–midwife relationship.
- Orchestration of environment.

removed from the equation, only 16.9% of women having first babies and 30.1% of women having a second or subsequent baby, could be classified as having a 'normal birth'. This study shrinks the domain of the midwife as 'guardian of the normal' and raises rhetorical questions about how we have failed in our guardianship (Beech 1997).

Any efforts to promote woman-centred maternity services need to be mindful of the social and cultural influences that hamper the acceptance of midwifery's potential role in society and health-care reforms. As identified by Raymond De Vries, confirmations of the value of midwifery need to be explored alongside 'new understandings of the forces that prevent the wisdom of midwifery from being realized' (De Vries 1996, p. 181). This is particularly evident in countries where the hegemony of private obstetrics operates at every level of the systems and ideology that control policy decision-making and public consciousness (Arney 1982). For example, in Australia, there is evidence identifying high intervention rates associated with private obstetric care (Roberts, Tracy and Peat 1999) and substantial costs associated with the initiation of a cascade of obstetric interventions (Tracy and Tracy 2003). In spite of this evidence, there are few signs of any radical changes in public health funding to include midwives as lead maternity care providers for low-risk women. In Australia, there is a long history of government policies that prioritize medical responsibility for pregnancy and birth, with structures that maximize economic benefit to the medical profession, in part, through maintenance of the subordination of midwives (Willis 1983). This compounds the challenge of developing the collaborative relationships that are necessary for introducing new models of care that increase midwives' visibility and contribution (Brodie 2002). While many obstetricians have applauded the concept of midwifery autonomy and have appreciated the scientific basis of its benefits, they have been unwilling to collaborate.

The process of understanding and addressing how such power imbalances affect women's experiences of maternity care is a challenge for the profession of midwifery. If midwives are to develop skills in questioning the status quo of the current policies and organization of maternity care, there needs to be a clear understanding of the potential role of midwifery leadership in transforming and enabling a different culture in the workplace.

THE GUARDIANSHIP ROLE OF TRANSFORMATIONAL MIDWIFERY LEADERS

A major leadership strategy for changing the culture of the birthing service was introduced by one of us (PB) when employed as a manager in a major Sydney hospital. Whenever a new group of midwifery students or medical staff started a rotation to the birthing suite, Pat would invite them to a welcome session and talk through the principles of promoting a woman-centred birthing culture. This would involve discussion along the lines listed in Box 10.4.

According to Avolio (1996), transformational change in organizations requires an outright 'attack' on the foundations of systems in order to abandon what is no longer working, while also providing some clear direction to pursue new initiatives. This process of abandonment and identifying future direction requires a higher-level leadership of the type known as 'transformational leadership' (Avolio 1996). We suggest that the notion of transformational leadership

---

Box 10.4   Promoting woman centred birthing territory with new staff

- Part of orientation for all new staff – medical and midwifery.
- Manager makes everyone feel welcome and includes all in setting the culture.
- Spelling out the 'ground rules' of being in a collaborative team.
- Expectations of all staff to be sensitive to individual woman's needs, particularly around privacy and respect.
- Expectations of sensitivity towards each other.
- 'Talking up' the shared benefits of satisfied women and families.
- Woman-centred care as part of professional interests and decision making.
- Reminding everyone of the profound long-term consequences and memories of this experience for women and their families.

sits comfortably with the guardianship role required of midwifery leaders.

Transformational leadership sees two or more individuals engaged in interactive processes that bring about increasing motivation and aspiration with an emphasis on progress, achievement and relationship (Rosener 1990). Leaders who possess transformational characteristics have the capacity to be innovative and creative and to bring into existence new structures, systems and processes, while continually raising their own and others' level of motivation and enthusiasm to succeed. This is what Anne-Marie Rafferty (1995) has referred to as 'the politics of optimism', whereby leaders influence change in a concerted way by 'talking up' the issue, putting a positive and palatable angle on the message that followers find appealing and appropriate.

Transformational leaders are characteristically democratic, participative and people oriented (Burns 1978). They engage in an 'interactive' leadership style that encourages others to transform their own self-interest into the interest of the group, through concern for the broader goal (Rosener 1990). They encourage participation, share power and information, enhance other people's self-worth and infuse others with excitement about their work.

Within the predominantly female profession of midwifery it is worth considering leadership styles that have been identified as particularly appealing to women. Eva Cox (1996) has written about women's uneasy relationship with leadership. She makes a plea for moving away from narrow definitions of leadership and for feminist ways of leading with an emphasis on power sharing:

> 'The onus of responsibility can be legitimately shared in ways which give us credit for skills and recognize diversity without hierarchy. Sharing the burdens and responsibilities also means sharing the fun of being effective.' (Cox 1996 p. 256)

It has been suggested that, among other things, women value caring, being involved, helping, being responsible, making intuitive decisions and forming networks rather than hierarchies (Kirner and Rayner 1999). It has also been argued that women are prepared to negotiate rather than argue, admit mistakes, share the credit and utilize highly effective social and interpersonal skills in building those networks (Rosener 1990; Cox 1996). This poses significant challenges for midwifery guardians, many of who will be women, as they seek to transform the culture of an organization constituted by significant numbers of powerful male doctors and service leaders. Such transformation requires a range of skills and competencies including emotional competence of the leader.

According to Raimond and Eden (1990) the emotional competence and capacity of a leader must be such that the strategic planning encouraged by the leader enhances the free flow of knowledge, ideas, information, values, beliefs and attitudes. A commitment to excellent communication is critical. These authors suggest that, in seeking this emotional involvement and commitment, essential energy and enthusiasm for change can be harnessed and channelled into the overall effort and shared vision (Raimond and Eden 1990). This resonates with our experiences in transforming the birthing culture. This involved huge amounts of energy and enthusiasm, which needed to be shared and perpetuated. Self-awareness and a level of maturity was also required, such that we needed to remain positive and 'on top' of things no matter the challenges or set backs we may have been experiencing.

Goleman et al (2001) cite research that shows an incontrovertible link between a leader's emotional maturity exemplified by such attributes as self-awareness and empathy, with explicit measures of success in achieving outcomes (Goleman, Boyatzis and McKee 2001). Extending his earlier work linking emotional intelligence with workplace culture (Goleman 1996), Goleman's more recent research indicates that the capacity to create work climates conducive to learning, information sharing, increasing trust and healthy risk taking between individuals, will be affected by the leader's mood and level of self-awareness and emotional intelligence (Goleman 2000). This in turn drives the moods, actions and outcomes of the entire group, team and/or organization (Goleman, Boyatzis and McKee 2001).

There is some evidence that leadership in the form of 'opinion leader education' is more effective in influencing changes to practice than that which might flow from audit feedback or research results (Taffinder 1995). With this in mind, it is important to determine what makes an 'opinion leader' in the health professions and what the attributes of a good leader are. In a profile of Edith Hillan, a midwifery leader in the UK, Barber (2000) has described how, in order for midwives to become leaders, they need to have a good grasp of the profession and the wider context in which it functions. Barber identifies how Hillan has called for universities, employers and professional organizations to jointly provide continuing education programs for current and future leaders of the profession, stressing that leaders need to be identified, supported, developed and encouraged (Barber 2000). In considering Hillan's notion of 'professional champions' in midwifery (Barber 2000), it is clear that such champions will need to emerge from a profession that has acquired significant levels of education and knowledge. Any practice development initiatives must also include attention directed at raising the quality of education at both the under graduate and postgraduate level for midwives.

Some specific skills related to leading and sustaining organizational change that we have learnt from midwifery leaders are identified in Box 10.5.

The next section in this chapter identifies how the principles of this style of leadership can be employed in creative strategies to promote woman-centred birthing territory and midwifery guardianship. We will draw on first hand examples of our experiences in various publicly funded maternity services.

REFORMING MATERNITY SERVICES – GUIDING PRINCIPLES

An understanding of, and commitment to, the philosophical principles of 'primary health-care' (World Health Organization 1986; Wass 1994) provides the ideal conceptual framework on which to base reforms in maternity services. Since the Declaration of Alma-Ata in 1978, primary health-care principles have influenced all World Health Organization policies. In relation to maternity services this means an approach that:

- addresses issues related to equity and access;
- encompasses determinants of health such as the influence of culture, education and income;

> **Box 10.5   Midwifery leadership skills when managing change**
>
> - Provision of clear, consistent, easy to understand information and rationale for changes.
> - A realistic timeframe that allows adequate time for people to process, adjust and prepare.
> - Willingness to listen to arguments against the idea and discuss them further.
> - Commitment to the vision with an awareness and willingness to change if intolerable complications ensue.
> - Capacity to manage minor fallout and move on.
> - Flexibility and a willingness to modify plans and approaches.
> - Awareness that 100% achievement of change is rare.
> - Establishment of a support team that include other leaders and managers who are committed to the same plan, goals and outcomes.
> - Ensuring that all stakeholders remain focused – played out in good chairing and recording of meetings.
> - Education programs to support professional development and change.

- develops services based on need that are affordable, sustainable and evidence-based;
- promotes community participation in all aspects of the development, implementation and evaluation of services;
- encourages the development of community based services;
- fosters collaboration, continuity of care and integrated services;
- uses appropriate technology;
- encourages self-reliance and the empowerment of community members.

These foundations underpin the reorganization of maternity services around a social model of birth (Kitzinger 2000; Kirkham 2003) and potentially restore the midwife to the rightful position in the community as the main provider of maternity care for the majority of women (Kaufmann 2002). In so doing, improved public health and long-term health gain, key outcomes of the new public health agenda (Downe 2001; Newburn 2001) could arguably be realized. This will only occur if midwives are able to practise to their full capacity, providing continuity of care, and maximizing women's capacity to labour and birth physiologically without unwarranted and costly intervention (Downe 2001).

A primary health-care approach to developing maternity services focuses on shifting the majority of maternity services into the community. We suggest that midwives are only able to facilitate a social model of birth if they [re]claim a style of working that is both physically and philosophically based in the community. It is ultimately questionable whether midwifery *can* flourish within the hegemony of fragmented, hospital systems that stifle the ability to practise 'woman-centred care' in a way that enriches the potential for women, and therefore their families and communities, to be more powerful.

ESTABLISHING MIDWIFERY CONTINUITY OF CARE

There is an imperative to enable situations in which women receive continuity of care from midwives who they know and trust if they are to feel 'safe' – physically, emotionally, spiritually and culturally – around birth. A growing body of evidence suggests that midwifery continuity of care makes a difference to women's experiences in terms of 'keeping birth normal' and promoting women's satisfaction with their experiences (Benjamin, Walsh and Taub 2001; Sandall, Davies and Warwick 2001; Page et al 2001; Homer, Davis and Cooke 2002). However, a note of caution about how 'continuity of care' and 'one-to-one' midwifery is enacted in some settings has been raised by Sheila Kitzinger (2005). She cites research in a UK hospital with a policy of one-to-one midwifery where 20 women were video-recorded during labour (Harris 2002). During these labours, 108 professional caregivers went in and out of the room and midwives spent only 15% of their time sitting alongside women and engaging with them. Kitzinger suggests there is lip service to continuity of care and that most midwifery care remains fragmented.

The Albany Midwifery Group Practice in south east London is held up as an example of caseload practice where a woman's primary midwife follows her across the interface of community and hospital arenas through pregnancy, labour and birth and the early weeks of new motherhood

(Reed 2002a, 2002b; Lester 2004). An evaluation of the Albany Midwifery Practice made comparisons with other midwifery group practices employed by Kings Health-care Trust in London and identified that 'the Albany practice was very successful at facilitating normality in pregnancy and birth' (Sandall et al 2001). Significant differences in outcomes were reported in terms of increased satisfaction for women; normal vaginal birth; home birth and breastfeeding rates; with reduced rates of induction; caesarean section; use of pharmacological pain relief; and perineal trauma (Sandall et al 2001).

An Australian model that aimed to replicate the Albany model, the Northern Women's Community Midwifery Project (NWCMP) has similar features, in that the midwives:

- are community based in a publicly funded model;
- cover a geographical area of extreme socio-economic deprivation;
- offer booking visits and a 36-week visit in the woman's home;
- run antenatal and postnatal groups;
- offer home birth as an option to all women with uncomplicated pregnancies.
- work with women of 'all risk'

Preliminary evaluations of the NWCMP (Nixon, Byrne and Church 2003) suggest similar positive outcomes for women and midwives as those identified in the evaluation of the Albany Midwifery Practice (Sandall et al 2001).

It is possible that the success of the Albany Midwives and the NWCMP lies in the fact that they provide a social model of midwifery care, one that sees bringing women together in groups as a crucial strategy to develop a forum where they can learn from each other and develop friendships and support networks (Leap 1991, 2004). As suggested by Mavis Kirkham, 'linking women with others makes them stronger' (Kirkham 1986, p. 47). Where the focus of antenatal groups centres on antenatal care as well as education and support, significant improvements in outcomes have been identified in disadvantaged communities in the USA (Schindler Rising 1998; Ickovics et al 2003), including a reduction in social isolation, prematurity and low birth weight babies. In models that promote support networks in the community, the locus of control is shifted away from health professionals and institutions and thus women are more able to take up powerful positions in their lives.

Practical considerations when setting up and supporting the development of midwifery group practices have been explored by several authors (Page 1995; Warwick 1996; Page, Cooke and Percival 2000; Homer, Brodie and Leap 2008). These texts describe experiences where midwives are able to engage with women in a rewarding process of transforming birth culture. Nowhere is this more apparent than where women are able to choose to give birth at home.

PROMOTING HOME BIRTH

The rationale to support publicly funded home birth was demonstrated recently in a large, landmark study in North America (Johnson and Davis 2005) that demonstrated a reduction in medical interventions and improved outcomes for women choosing to give birth at home. In many Western countries, homebirth has been shown to be a safe option for a carefully selected group of women (Tyson 1991; Campbell and Macfarlane 1994; Anderson and Murphy 1995; Ackermann-Leibrich et al 1996; Davies et al 1996; Wiegers, Keirse and van der Zee 1996; Chamberlain, Wraight and Crowley 1997; Olsen 1997; Murphy and Fullerton 1998; Olsen and Jewell 1998). Similar findings have been demonstrated in Australia and New Zealand (Crotty et al 1990; Woodcock et al 1990; Gulbransen, Hilton and McKay 1997; New Zealand Ministry of Health 1999–2002) although poor outcomes have been associated with women with risk associated pregnancies, such as twins and breeches, opting

---

Box 10.6 Promoting community based, midwifery continuity of care

- Addressing primary health-care principles.
- A social model of birth.
- Promoting friendships and support networks among women.
- Shifting the locus of control to women.
- 'Groups not classes' (Leap 1991, 2004).
- Public funding, including for home birth.

---

for birth at home in Australia (Bastian, Keirse and Lancaster 1998).

While women in New Zealand and the UK have the opportunity to give birth within publicly funded maternity services, in Australia, the development of such options is in its infancy. Community-based midwifery programs, which incorporate homebirth options in a publicly funded health-care system, have been successfully implemented in both Western Australia (Thiele and Thorogood 1997; Thorogood, Thiele and Hyde 2002) and in the previously mentioned, NWCMP in South Australia (Nixon et al 2003), with safe outcomes for both mothers and babies and high levels of satisfaction for women and midwives.

The first publicly funded home birth service in New South Wales started in late 2005 from St George Hospital (SGH), Kogarah in southern Sydney. This was a result of several years of negotiation and planning at local and state health service levels, particularly around securing insurance for midwives employed in the health service. Support from certain obstetricians at SGH and collaboration with local home birth support networks were crucial elements of success in these negotiations. The home birth service at SGH is embedded in an existing service – it is 'another option' offered to all women receiving birth centre care from midwives already working in a caseload practice model. This is an important consideration in terms of introducing an accessible, sustainable model that is part of mainstream service provision. Other than for evaluation, no extra funding needed to be secured to introduce the home birth option and the risk of 'death by pilot project' – the clawing back of additional funds – was avoided. There are many other lessons to be shared in reflecting on our experience of being involved in the development of this service. Some examples are seen in Box 10.7.

Given the evidence that planned home birth is just as safe as birth in hospital for the majority of women who have uncomplicated pregnancies (Olsen and Jewell 1998), the promotion and support of homebirth as a mainstream option for women, has to be a major tactic in promoting physiological birth and woman-centred birth territory. Resistance to such a proposal

---

Box 10.7 Setting up a new publicly funded home birth service

- Full involvement on the steering committee of women, organizations who promote home birth, and a range of health professionals representing: independent midwives; midwives employed in the public health system; obstetricians; paediatricians; GPs; the ambulance service.
- The development of an information leaflet for women and their families with positive messages about the safety of home birth and relevant websites.
- Embedding the model in an existing caseload practice model, so that it is seen as another option to offer all

women accessing this service (as opposed to a separate service that only women 'in the know' can access).
- Mentoring of midwives who have little or no experience of home birth by midwives with extensive experience of home birth.
- Monitoring of requests from women who are unable to access the service due to living outside the catchment area, so that a need can be identified and the service developed elsewhere.

---

is enshrined in the discourse of contemporary maternity services. With this in mind, the House of Commons Select Committee on Maternity Services (2003) proposed that all midwives, GPs or obstetricians should be enabled to attend a home birth during their training in order to challenge their prejudices and familiarize them with the promotion of normal birth (House of Commons 2003). Anecdotal evidence suggests that attending a birth at home has a significant effect on the practice of both midwives and doctors in terms of giving them an insight into the profound nature of birth and the power of physiology.

Public awareness about the safety of home birth also needs to be addressed in any strategy to promote woman-centred birthing territory. As identified by the Albany Midwifery Practice where over 50% of women give birth at home, it is possible to support people to come to the realization that home birth is a safe option, even where they would never have considered it before. This practice has been able to show that where known midwives engage with women and their supporters throughout pregnancy, in particular during a home visit in late pregnancy, and where decision making about the place of birth is reserved for labour, home birth is a safe option for the majority of women. Inevitably this also leads to a significant decrease in operative birth and medical interventions (Reed 2002a,b).

Similar principles to those surrounding the promotion of home birth need to be applied in the promotion of birth centres. A useful resource when exploring this is a book edited by Mavis

Kirkham, *Birth Centres – A Social Model for Maternity Care* (Kirkham 2003). Within over 20 examples of very different birth centre settings in different countries, the same message emerges: the philosophy and scale of birth centres enable an environment where midwives can develop skills and confidence to support and trust women's ability to give birth without intervention. What is described over again is the midwifery art of 'being with' women in labour and 'working with' pain (Leap 1997; Leap and Anderson 2004).

THE PROMOTION OF PHYSIOLOGY: 'BEING WITH' WOMEN IN PAIN

It has been suggested that the key to promoting physiological birth is directly linked to midwives' ability to be with women in pain and resist the temptation to 'rescue' them through offering 'pain relief' (Leap and Anderson 2004). Creating a culture where all members of staff understand the value of an approach described as 'working with' pain, rather than one of 'pain relief' (Leap 1997) is a strategy that we both use in the development of our own birthing environments in public hospitals. This often means simple actions such as reassuring all those not involved in a woman's care, including support people and other staff, that her highly audible vocalizing is indeed a positive sign of good progress, something to be welcomed rather than something requiring intervention or assistance. This is only possible if there is a degree of trust of the midwife's clinical judgment and recognition of the important relationship that exists between the woman and her midwife. In addition to this we prioritize regular opportunities for multidisciplinary learning and discussion about care of women in labour and issues regarding the use of analgesia.

At these sessions staff can explore their feelings and attitudes when being alongside women whose labours are progressing well but who are vocalizing and expressing doubts about whether they can cope with the pain. The temptation to prejudge the midwife's clinical practices and decision making about a woman's pain relief must also be resisted. As identified in a report by the Royal College of Obstetricians and Gynaecologists (Maclean, Stones and Thornton 2001) it is important for maternity service staff to explore their feelings of discomfort around being with women in pain in labour, particularly in terms of how they might influence the choices women make to use narcotics and epidurals. Consideration of the evidence in Box 10.8 provides a springboard for discussion regarding how best to approach being with women in pain.

THE '36–WEEK HOME VISIT'

When considering strategies to encourage women and their birth supporters to explore the benefits of labour without pharmacological 'pain relief' it is worth considering an important study carried out by Joy Kemp (2003) describing midwives', women's and their birth partners' experiences of a '36-week home visit'. The initiative was described as:

'. . .an alternative model of authoritative knowledge, one which acknowledged a role for intervention and technology but placed as central a philosophy of birth as a physiological, transformational and socio-cultural event.' (Kemp 2003, p. 4)

In her research, Joy Kemp (2003) identified a range of productive activities involved in carrying out the 36-week home visit. These included the following practicalities shown in Box 10.9.

Kemp's (2003) study portrayed the 36-week birth talk as an integral part of the ongoing dialogue and relationship of mutual trust that occurs between a woman and her midwife, throughout pregnancy, where the same midwife or midwives are going to be with the woman during labour. The concept is thus directly related to continuity of care that includes an intrapartum component. It is also one element of a midwifery model that aims to focus on birth as a social, rather than a technocratic, event (Kitzinger 2000) and further assists in the construction of woman-centred birthing territory.

COLLEGIALITY AND INTERDISCIPLINARY SUPPORT

All of the strategies to promote physiological birth that have been addressed so far in this chapter will flourish in an environment where

---

Box 10.8   Evidence to inform discussion about pain in labour

- Women's satisfaction with their experience of birth is not related to analgesia (Morgan et al 1982; Hodnett 2002).
- The most powerful influence on a woman's feeling of satisfaction is the attitudes of her caregivers (Hodnett 2002).
- Although almost all women will describe the pain of labour as extremely severe, those who used non-pharmacological methods of pain relief are less likely to complain that they had unbearable pain (Chamberlain, Wraight and Steer 1993).
- Epidurals increase the risk of instrumental birth (Roberts et al 1999; Elzschig, Lieberman and Camman 2003) and are not associated with increased satisfaction.
- There are good reasons to avoid giving labouring women pethidine and the majority of women find it dulls their capacity to express pain, rather than relieve it (Olofsson, Ekblom and Ekman-Ordeberg 1996; Heelbeck 1999).
- Culturally diverse groups of women have described childbirth as a difficult, yet empowering, experience leading to a sense of achievement and feeling of pride in their ability to cope with intense pain (Halldorsdottir and Karlsdottir 1996; Lundgren and Dahlberg 1998; Niven and Murphy-Black 2000; Callister et al 2003).

Box 10.9   Promoting physiological birth through a 36-week home visit

- Involving family members planning to be involved in support in labour and in the early days following birth, with practical suggestions for how this might take place.
- Discussions about approaches to being with women in pain in labour without rushing to take away pain and to ensure that physiology is promoted.

- The use of photographs to encourage discussion about normal birth.
- Information to reduce premature admission to hospital in labour.
- Decision-making about choice about place of birth in labour.

there is collegiality and high quality mutual support for practitioners. Developing a supportive culture is about breaking down hierarchical barriers, enabling safe situations for all practitioners to share their uncertainty as well as their expertise, and recognizing different expertise and complementary roles. Such an approach also depends on the most powerful groups – doctors – relinquishing some of their power. Power cannot be given, it can only be taken and this process involves mutual sensitivity to the dynamics and potential pitfalls surrounding collaboration on the part of both parties.

There is great benefit in organizing interprofessional interaction. We have both worked in units where, most days at lunchtime there is some form of interdisciplinary get together or 'in-service' in the meeting room. This could be any of the initiatives shown in Box 10.10.

In our experience, regular coming together for events such as those described in the box below, change the way that midwives and doctors interact within their inter-professional milieu. This has been noted elsewhere. In units where multidisciplinary efforts are activated to reduce caesarean sections, success may well be about raising consciousness and awareness about

issues and philosophical approaches, plus a concerted effort from all disciplines, rather than specific strategies per se – such as locking all fetal monitors in the cupboard and requiring a written explanation for their use. It seems that pulling together, a commitment to evidence-based practice, one-to-one support from midwives during labour, managing change and fostering goodwill are important strategies in reducing interference in labour and improving outcomes for women (Ontario Women's Health Council 2002).

The successful implementation of new models of care, that place the woman at the centre of care and increase the autonomy of midwives, may well be dependent upon inter-professional trust and collaboration (Brodie 1996). Collaboration in maternity care presents opportunities to improve care for women. In settings where new models of care and effective collaborative relationships between midwives and obstetricians are developed simultaneously, a number of potentially beneficial effects have been suggested. These include the factors listed in Box 10.11.

Collaboration is an emergent process rather than an outcome; thus, collaborations move from 'under organized systems' in which all

Box 10.10   Interdisciplinary initiatives

- A monthly perinatal mortality meeting where midwives as well as doctors present cases for review.
- Interesting case reviews – led by midwives, doctors or students on a rotational basis.
- Consensus guidelines for practice development – evidence-based and incorporating woman centred approaches to practice.

- Student project presentations – students are encouraged to present their projects to all staff.
- Topic based review of putting evidence into practice – guided discussion sessions.
- Regular emergency practice drills.

Box 10.11   The rationale for interdisciplinary collaboration

- Where midwifery care 'follows the woman' regardless of the existence or development of 'risk' factors (McCourt, Page and Hewison 1998), collaboration with medical specialists and others is essential.
- Maintenance of midwifery as a central component in the care of *all* women (Hodnett 2005).
- Development of autonomous midwifery skills and confidence (Page et al 2000).

- Maintenance of the integrity of the role and range of skills of the midwife – not 'sub specializing' (Page et al 2000).
- Improved relationships and experiences – for women, midwives, doctors (Brodie 1996b; Homer et al 2001).
- The potential to improve clinical outcomes (Homer et al 2001).

---

stakeholders act independently, to more tightly organized relationships characterized by concerted decision making (Gray 1989). Gray's work portrays the dynamic and forever changing domain of collaboration that is a part of the everyday relationships and organizational culture of maternity care. If collaboration is successful, new solutions emerge that no single party could have envisaged or enacted (Gray 1999). Applied to maternity service provision and effective care, such a process requires deliberate focus, articulation, understanding and the leadership of professionals. It is our view that while collaboration as part of routine care is not made explicit, its powerful potential for improved decision making and better outcomes will not be realized. Moreover it may work to hide what may simply be 'cooperation' by midwives who are almost always in a subservient and subordinate position within the inter-professional relationship.

A greater understanding of factors that enhance or inhibit health-care providers' capacity to work together collaboratively, and the inherent benefits of doing so, may be of benefit. We both have experience of working in situations where the institutionalized power of an obstetrician was a significant and insurmountable barrier to truly effective collaboration and therefore any progress in expanding midwifery models of care. In contrast we have worked in a maternity service where there is a serious commitment from midwifery and obstetric leaders to explore, analyse and change the prevailing culture [of medical dominance] and move towards a more collaborative approach to service provision (Everitt et al 1995).

In the experience of one of us (PB) involved in implementing the team midwifery model of care that was evaluated by Homer et al (2001), the development of trust between midwives and obstetricians was a crucial element in both the development and subsequent sustainability of the model. Midwives were required to work alone or in pairs as autonomous practitioners based in a community setting, separate from the mainstream hospital services and personnel. They made clinical decisions under their own responsibility and scope of practice, and referred and consulted with obstetricians and others as necessary. While the nature of the study made it impossible to measure cause and effect, it is feasible to assert that the collaboration itself was a critical factor in the impressive outcomes for the women experiencing this care [4% reduction in caesarean section rate; women more satisfied; and reduced costs] (Homer, Davis and Brodie 2000, 2001b,c; Homer, Matha et al. 2001). This collaborative professional relationship was based on a clear understanding of roles and boundaries of practice, a focus on woman-centred care and a growing level of respect and trust that developed between midwives and obstetricians, which continues to the present day (Homer et al 2008).

The model that we developed in Australia, the 'St George Outreach Maternity Program' (STOMP) was set up with a deliberate focus on collaboration between midwives and obstetricians as part of a community based maternity service available to women of all levels of risk. Outcomes of the randomized controlled trial at St George involving 1089 women demonstrated a significant difference in the caesarean section rate between the groups, 13.3% in the STOMP group and 17.8% in the control group. This difference was maintained after controlling for known contributing factors to caesarean section. Women receiving STOMP care were more satisfied and costs associated with the new model were less than for standard care (Homer, Davis and Brodie, 2000; Homer et al 2001b,c).

In our experience, through the provision of a positive professional working environment, the practices of midwives and others may be enhanced, which in turn may improve the outcomes of the care provided to women. Changing culture in mainstream maternity service provision requires midwives and doctors to come together and re-evaluate how they interact and work together. This can be enhanced by willingness and a degree of professional generosity that is rare and desperately needed in traditional settings (Kirkham 1996; Kirkham and Stapleton 1999).

THE IMPORTANCE OF TRUST IN COLLABORATIVE RELATIONSHIPS

When midwives and doctors collaborate effectively there are exchanges of essential ideas and information. This exchange of ideas and information can only occur if there is a sharing of power and responsibility along with recognition of the need for occupational autonomy. In contemporary maternity services, provision of such 'sharing' of power' in essence means that doctors must give up some of their power. This requires a sophisticated level of mutual trust.

There is a growing body of literature that assists in explaining why and how trust is an essential element of collaborative relationships and organizational effectiveness (Limerick and Cunnington 1993). In any relationship, trust evolves and changes over time. Not all relationships develop fully and many professional relationships in health-care services do not advance beyond a very preliminary and superficial perception of trust.

What emerges from an understanding of trust is that without it, relationships cannot develop. Without a relationship there is no possibility of collaboration. Critically, without collaborative trusting relationships the potential to improve health-care and maternity care in particular is severely limited.

In a study of the development of a team midwifery program (Brodie 1996) the basic social process underpinning each team midwife's experience of her new role was trust. This manifested in trusting relationships with both women and other professionals:

- Trust built over time as a result of positive social and professional interactions between individuals and the work of the team and the organization.
- Trust enabled the team midwives to '...open up and let go of the previous role and believe in women and ourselves more'.
- Trust also enhanced the team midwives' ability to be with women and advocate for them.

In our experience, a major strategy to promote trust is bringing together midwives in 'teams' or group practices at least once a week, to discuss their experiences and support each other. As identified by Jane Sandall (1997), regular coming together is an essential component of successful midwifery continuity of care models and frequent meetings play a major role in the avoidance of 'burn out' and isolation.

The culture of midwifery is strengthened where leaders organize to support midwives in coming together to tell stories about their practice and experiences:

> 'A story tells more than its tale. It speaks of context and of values. Listeners absorb the story through a web of their own view of the world and by links with their own stories... Stories reveal important aspects of midwives' work and their careful examination may open up new dimensions in which we can usefully be with women.' (Kirkham 1997, p. 183)

There are good reasons to encourage situations where midwives can get together to tell stories about their practice. Kim Walker (1995) suggests that the value of story telling arises from the opportunities to articulate, but then critique, the complexity and diversity of clinical practice. He proposes a two way process where 'our lives and experiences are not merely reflected in stories: they are instead, actually created by and through them' (Walker 1995, p. 156). As Hannah Williams (2003) identified when observing and interviewing midwives in

> **Box 10.12 The importance of 'coming together' regularly**
>
> - Building trust and support.
> - Breaking down hierarchical relationships.
> - Clarity about roles and responsibilities.
> - Working out flexible, 'on call' arrangements.
> - Sharing knowledge and skills.
> - Story telling to promote understanding and wonder about birth.

> **Box 10.13 Changes to birthing space within budget**
>
> - Setting aside a space for normal labour and birth, removing the bed and refurbishing it to look like the sort of room seen in a play centre 'soft room'.
> - Donation of furniture, furnishings and paint by local stores (recognition of contributions can be displayed discreetly).
> - Fund raising for birthing pools, bean bags, birthing balls, floor mattresses, hanging ropes, squatting bars in every room.
> - Avoiding white – warm, dark colours for all furniture and walls (including pools).
> - Plenty of soft surfaces with cushions for all – including midwives – to rest on while waiting for labour to unfold.
> - The use of screens in front of doors and to cordon off private areas within rooms.

a London birth centre, almost all narratives began with, 'I had a lady who...' Williams suggests that this is the midwifery equivalent of 'Once upon a time...' She concluded that midwifery stories play a major role in developing an occupational culture in which the physiology of birth is admired and respected, where women's strength in giving birth is acknowledged and where midwives are encouraged to develop new skills (Williams 2003).

CHANGING THE PHYSICAL ENVIRONMENT

We have left to last a short discussion on the most obvious aspect of creating woman-centred birth territory – changing the physical environment. Even where new maternity units are built, it is rare that any radical changes in architecture and design are implemented. Brand new birthing rooms may have equipment hidden behind sliding doors and there may be some attempt at 'homeliness' with furniture and fittings, but the bed-centred starkness of twentieth century hospital birthing rooms persists.

Whether it is a case of planning a new maternity unit or making changes to an existing one, midwives can play an important role in changing people's thinking if they make sure they are on planning committees as well as the organizations that set standards for hospital facilities. Persuading people to think 'outside of the square' about design in relation to birthing spaces is a project that is best approached by forming a group of like-minded people who will enthuse others. In our experience, finding an architect in a university with an interest in designing facilities that promote healing and

wellbeing is an excellent catalyst. This can open the opportunity to engage in an action research project where all key players are involved in designing a space that is comfortable for all involved, but importantly, a space that promotes physiology for labouring women. Underpinning this, for all involved, needs to be an essential respect for the swirling, neuro-hormonal cascades of normal labour and an understanding of the potential effect of environment on these (Odent (1984, 1992). Again we return to education initiatives to raise awareness about the issues that are explored throughout this book.

CONCLUSION

Any exploration of how the notions of 'birth territory' and 'midwifery guardianship' are carried out in maternity systems raises issues that reach beyond the questioning of individual midwives' practice and the environment in which that is enacted. The opportunity for midwives to stand back and think about such issues forces us to confront challenges that threaten to extinguish midwifery in a culture of technocratic hegemony dominated by obstetric thinking (Davis-Floyd and Sargent 1997; Murphy-Lawless 1998). The tension between addressing the necessary shift away from this technocratic culture and the need for collaborative relationships will no doubt continue to challenge all involved in maternity care.

As we have discussed in this chapter, the development and continuation of collaborative partnerships between maternity care providers is a critical factor in the successful implementation of new models of care that improve experiences and outcomes for women (Homer et al 2001c). Crucially, understanding the need for recognition of, and respect for, the existence of the unique and separate identities of midwife and obstetrician (Hardy, Lawrence and Phillips 1999), will be integral to the success of any collaboration in maternity care. Such understandings will be crucial as collaborative processes begin to develop and the inevitable explorations of competing and conflicting interests and power differentials unfold.

In fulfilling our midwifery guardianship role, there is an imperative to respond to Sheila Kitzinger's urgent challenge for all involved to explore how we may come together and enable a social model of childbirth:

'This is a challenge for all of us, nationally and internationally, not only for our sakes, but for our daughters, and their daughters after them. If, through fear and ignorance, we neglect our heritage and allow technocracy to take over, woman-centred childbirth may be lost forever.' (Kitzinger 2000, p. 250)

Conceptualizing midwifery as a profession that must urgently capitalize on its inherent qualities, attributes and potential is an important step in responding to this challenge. Starting with the language we use, the importance of articulating the philosophical underpinnings of our practice is a crucial step towards shaping a new culture in maternity service provision. As we have identified, primary health-care principles need to underpin a community development approach to reforming maternity services

that are equitable, accessible, sustainable and community-based. Our midwifery guardianship role requires us to have a vision of how this might happen so that we may articulate the way forward, share our experiences and knowledge, tell our stories and provide theory from which to act.

Ultimately, the nexus of the necessary recovery of midwifery lies in the hearts and minds of midwives themselves and in their ability to engage with women:

'Only when women and midwives build a strong and supportive sisterhood which enables women to give birth in their own way, in their own time, and in their own place, can midwifery be re-born.' (Kitzinger 1995, p. x).

We have shared some of our experiences of engaging with women in this chapter and have identified the importance of developing midwifery continuity of care models that include bringing women together in groups and promoting home birth as an option for the majority of women. We have also discussed the importance of creating a culture of 'being with' women in pain in labour as a major strategy to promote physiological birth.

In attempting a pragmatic exploration of ways of narrowing the gap between the 'ideal' and the 'real', this chapter has explored how the midwife's guardianship role in promoting woman-centred birthing territory involves infinitely more than physical changes to the environment and a series of techniques used in labour. It involves the raising of consciousness at every level – in communities, between practitioners and in our institutions, health services and governments – in order to build systems and services that nurture the potential of birth to transform lives and strengthen women, their families, communities and societies.

References

Ackermann-Leibrich U, Voegeli T, Gunter-Wint K et al 1996 Home versus hospital deliveries: Follow up study of matched pairs for procedures and outcome. British Medical Journal 313: 1313–1318.

ACM 2002 ACM Standards for the Accreditation of 3 year Bachelor of Midwifery Programs. Australian College of Midwives, Melbourne.

ACM 2004 Australian College of Midwives Philosophy Statement. Australian College of Midwives, Canberra. Available on website: www.midwives.org.au

Anderson R, Murphy P 1995 Outcomes of 11,788 planned homebirths attended by certified nurse-midwives. A retrospective descriptive study. Journal of Nurse-Midwifery 40: 483–492.

ANMC 2006 ANMC National Competency Standards for the Midwife. Australian Nurses and Midwives Council, Canberra.

Arney WR 1982 Power and the profession of obstetrics. The University of Chicago Press, Chicago.

Avolio B 1996 What's all the Karping about down under? In: K Parry (Ed). Leadership research and practice; emerging themes and new challenges. Pitman, Victoria, pp. 3–15.

Barber T 2000 Leaders of midwifery: Professor Edith Hillan. Royal College of Midwives Journal 3: 114–115.

Bastian H 1992 Confined, managed and delivered: The language of obstetrics. British Journal of Obstetrics and Gynaecology 99: 92–93.

Bastian H, Keirse M, Lancaster P 1998 Perinatal death associated with planned homebirth in Australia: Population based study. British Medical Journal 317: 384–388.

Beech B 1997 Normal birth: Does it exist? Association for Improvements in the Maternity Services (AIMS) Journal 9: 4–8.

Benjamin Y, Walsh D, Taub N 2001 A comparison of partnership caseload practice with conventional team midwifery care: Labour and birth outcomes. Midwifery 17: 234–240.

Brodie P 1996 Being with women: The experiences of Australian team midwives. Masters Thesis. University of Technology, Sydney, Unpublished thesis.

Brodie P 2002 Addressing the barriers to midwifery – Australian midwives speaking out. Journal of the Australian College of Midwives 15(3): 5–14.

Burns J 1978 Leadership. Harper and Row, New York.

Callister LC, Khalaf I, Semenic S et al 2003 The pain of childbirth: Perceptions of culturally diverse women. Pain Management in Nursing 4(4): 145–154.

Campbell R, Macfarlane A 1994 Where to be born? The debate and the evidence, 2nd edn. National Perinatal Epidemiology Unit.

Chamberlain G, Wraight A, Crowley P 1997 Home births: The report of the 1994 confidential enquiry by the National Birthday Trust Fund. Parthenon, Carnforth.

Chamberlain G, Wraight A, Steer P (Eds) 1993 Pain and its relief in childbirth: The results of a national survey conducted by the National Birthday Trust. Churchill Livingstone, Edinburgh.

Cox E 1996 Leading women. Random House, Sydney.

Crotty M, Ramsay A, Smart R, Chan A 1990 Planned homebirths in South Australia 1976–1987. Medical Journal of Australia 153: 664–671.

Davies J, Hey E, Reid W, Young G 1996 Prospective regional study of planned home births. Home Birth Study Steering Group. British Medical Journal 313: 1302–1306.

Davis-Floyd R 1994 The technocratic body: American childbirth as cultural expression. Social Science and Medicine 38: 1125–1140.

Davis-Floyd R 2001 The technocratic, humanistic and holistic paradigms of childbirth. International Journal of Gynaecology Obstetrics 75, S5–S23.

Davis-Floyd R, Sargent C 1997 Childbirth and authoritative knowledge: Cross cultural perspectives. University of California Press, Berkely, CA.

De Vries M 1996 Making midwives legal: Childbirth, medicine and the Law, 2nd edn. Ohio State University Press, Austin, TX.

Declercq E 1994 A cross-national analysis of midwifery politics: Six lessons for midwives. Midwifery 10(4): 232–237.

Downe S 2001 Making a difference: A strategy for health gain in maternity services. Midwifery Matters (Summer) 89: 26–27.

Downe S, McCormick C, Beech B 2001 Labour interventions associated with normal birth. British Journal of Midwifery 9(10): 602–606.

Elzschig HK, Lieberman ES, Camman WR 2003 Regional anaesthesia and analgesia for labor and delivery. New England Journal of Medicine 348: 319–332.

Everitt L, Barclay L, Chapman M et al 1995 St George Maternity Services Customer Satisfaction Research Project. St George Hospital and Community Services, Sydney.

Fahy K 1998 Being a midwife or doing midwifery. Australian College of Midwives Journal 11(2): June 11–16.

Flint C 1988 On the brink: Midwifery in Britain. In: S Kitzinger (Ed). The Midwife Challenge. Pandora, London, pp. 22–39.

Flint C 1993 Midwifery teams and caseloads. Butterworth-Heinemann, Oxford.

Goleman D 1996 Emotional intelligence. Bloomsbury, London.

Goleman D 2000 Leadership that gets results. Harvard Business Review, March–April, pp. 78–90.

Goleman D, Boyatzis R, McKee M 2001 Primal leadership: The hidden driver of great performance. Harvard Business Review 79(11 Special Issue): 42–52.

Gray B 1989 Collaborating. Jossey-Bass, San Francisco.

Gray B 1999 Theoretical perspectives on collaboration over the last decade: Looking back and looking forward. Sydney.

Guilliland K, Pairman S 1995 The midwifery partnership: A model for practice. Department of Nursing and Midwifery Monograph Series, Victoria University, Wellington, New Zealand.

Gulbransen G, Hilton J, McKay L 1997 Home birth in New Zealand 1973–1993: incidence and mortality. New Zealand Medical Journal 110: 87–89.

Halldorsdottir S, Karlsdottir SI 1996 Journeying through labour and delivery: perceptions of women who have given birth. Midwifery 12(2): 48–61.

Hardy C, Lawrence T, Phillips N 1999 Changing conversations, collective identity and inter-organizational collaboration. Collaboration Research and Practice Seminar: Academic and Executive Perspectives.

Harris M 2002 An investigation of labour ward care to inform the design of a computerised decision support system for the management of childbirth. University of Plymouth [Unpublished Doctoral thesis].

Hastie C 2005 How understanding semantics helps us be 'with women'. MIDIRS Midwifery Digest 15(4): 475–477.

Heelbeck L 1999 Administration of pethidine in labour. British Journal of Midwifery 7: 372–377.

Hewison A 1993 The language of labour: An examination of the discourses of childbirth. Midwifery 9: 225–234.

Hodnett ED 2002 Pain and women's satisfaction with the experience of childbirth: A systematic review. American Journal of Obstetrics and Gynaecology 186(5): S160–S172.

Hodnett ED 2005 Continuity of care givers during pregnancy and childbirth (Cochrane Review). Cochrane Database of Systematic Reviews, Issue 2, Oxford.

Homer C, Brodie P, Leap N 2008 Midwifery continuity of care: A practical guide. Elsevier (in press).

Homer C, Davis G, Brodie P 2000 What do women feel about community-based antenatal care? Australian and New Zealand Journal of Public Health 24(6): 590–595.

Homer C, Davis G, Brodie P et al 2001c Collaboration in maternity care: A randomised controlled trial comparing community-based continuity of care with standard hospital care. British Journal of Obstetrics and Gynaecology 108 (January): 16–22.

Homer C, Davis G, Cooke M 2002 Women's experiences of continuity of midwifery care in a randomised controlled trial in Australia. Midwifery 18(2): 102–112.

Homer C, Matha D, Jordan L, Wills J, Davis G 2001b Community-based continuity of midwifery care versus standard hospital care: A cost analysis. Australian Health Review 24(1): 85–93.

House of Commons 2003 House of Commons Select Committee on Maternity Services. HMSO, London.

Ickovics JR, Kershaw TS, Westdahl C et al 2003 Group prenatal care and preterm birth weight: Results from a two-site matched cohort study. Obstetrics and Gynecology 102: 1051–1057.

Johnson KC, Davis BA 2005 Outcomes of planned home births with certified professional midwives: Large prospective study in North America. British Medical Journal 330.

Katz-Rothman B 1996 Women, providers and control. Journal of Obstetrics, Gynaecology and Neonatal Nursing 25(3): 253–256.

Kaufmann T 2002 Midwifery and public health. MIDIRS Midwifery Digest, March (12 Supplement 1): S23–S26.

Kemp J 2003 Midwives', women's and their birth partners' experiences of the 36 week birth talk: A qualitative study. Unpublished thesis. The Florence Nightingale School of Nursing and Midwifery, Kings College London.

Kirkham M 1986 A feminist perspective in midwifery. In: C Webb (Ed). Feminist practice in women's health. John Wiley, Chichester, pp. 35–49.

Kirkham M 1996 Professionalization past and present: With women or with the powers that be? In: D Kroll (Ed). Midwifery care for the future: Meeting the challenge. Bailliere-Tindall, London, pp. 164–201.

Kirkham M 1997 Stories and childbirth. In: MJ Kirkham, ER Perkins (Eds). Reflections on midwifery. Bailliere Tindall, London, pp. 183–204.

Kirkham M 2000 The midwife/mother relationship. Macmillan, London.

Kirkham M 2003 Birth centres – A social model for maternity care. Books for Midwives, London.

Kirkham M, Stapleton H 1999 The culture of midwifery in the NHS in England. Journal of Advanced Nursing 30: 732–739.

Kirner J, Rayner M 1999 The women's power handbook. Penguin, London.

Kitzinger S 1995 Foreward by Sheila Kitzinger. In: M O'Conner (Ed). Birth tides: Turning towards home birth. Pandora, London.

Kitzinger S 2000 Rediscovering birth. Little Brown, Boston.

Kitzinger S 2005 The language of birth. MIDIRS Midwifery Digest 15(2), June: 209–210.

Leap N 1991 Helping you to make your own decisions – antenatal and postnatal groups in Deptford, SE London. VHS Video. Available from Birth International. www.birthinternational.com.au.

Leap N 1992 The power of words and the confinement of women: How language affects midwives' practice. Nursing Times 88(12): 60–61.

Leap N 1997 A midwifery perspective on pain in labour. Unpublished MSc Dissertation. South Bank University, London.

Leap N 2000 The less we do, the more we give. In: M Kirkham (Ed). The midwife–mother relationship. Macmillan, Basingstoke.

Leap N 2004 Journey to midwifery through feminism: A personal account. Chapter 13. In: M Stewart (Ed). Pregnancy, birth and maternity care: Feminist perspectives. London: Books for Midwives Press, pp. 185–200.

Leap N, Anderson T 2004 The role of pain and the empowerment of women. In: S Downe (Ed). Normal childbirth: Evidence and debate. Churchill Livingstone, Edinburgh.

Leap N, Hunter B 1993 The midwife's tale: An oral history from handywoman to professional midwife. Scarlet Press, Gateshead.

Lester A 2004 The argument for caseload midwifery. Midwifery Matters (103): Winter edition, 9–12.

Limerick D, Cunnington B 1993 Managing the new organization. Jossey-Bass, San Francisco.

Lundgren I, Dahlberg K 1998 Women's experience of pain during childbirth. Midwifery 14(2): 105–110.

Maclean A, Stones R, Thornton S 2001 Pain in obstetrics and gynaecology. Royal College of Obstetricians and Gynaecologists, London. (Recommendations accessible via RCOG website www.rcog.org.uk Page ID=441).

McCourt C, Page L, Hewison J 1998 Evaluation of one-to-one midwifery: Women's responses to care. Birth 25: 73–80.

Morgan BM, Bulpitt CJ, Clifton P, Lewis PJ 1982 Analgesia and satisfaction in childbirth. Lancet ii: 808–810.

Murphy P, Fullerton J 1998 Outcomes of intended home births in nurse-midwifery practice: A prospective descriptive study. Obstetrics and Gynecology 92: 461–470.

Murphy-Lawless J 1998 Reading birth and death. Cork University Press, Cork, Ireland.

New Zealand Ministry of Health (1999–2002) Reports on maternity: Maternity and newborn information. New Zealand Ministry of Health, Wellington.

Newburn M 2001 All Party Parliamentary Group on Maternity Care – A national service framework for maternity care. The Practising Midwife 4(2): 10–12.

Niven C, Murphy-Black T 2000 Memory for labor pain: A review of the literature. Birth 27(4): 244–253.

Nixon A, Byrne J, Church A 2003 The Community Midwives Project: An evaluation of the set-up of Northern Women's Community Midwives Project. June 1998–November 2000. Auspiced by Northern Metropolitan Community Health Services, South Australia. Adelaide: Northern Metropolitan Community Health Service, South Australia.

Odent M 1984 Birth re-born: What birth can and should be. Souvenir Press, London.

Odent M 1992 The nature of birth and breastfeeding. Bergin Garvey, Westport, CT.

Olofsson C, Ekblom A, Ekman-Ordeberg G 1996 Lack of analgesic effect of systematically administered morphine or pethidine on labour pain. British Journal of Obstetrics and Gynaecology 103: 968–972.

Olsen O 1997 Meta-analysis of the safety of homebirth. Birth 24: 4–13.

Olsen O, Jewell MD 1998 Home birth versus hospital birth (Cochrane Review). The Cochrane Library (Issue 3).

Ontario Women's Health Council 2002 Attaining and maintaining best practices in the use of caesarean sections. An analysis of four Ontario hospitals. Report of the Caesarean Section Working Group of the Women's Health Council: www.womenshealth-council.com.

Page L 1993 Redefining the midwife's role: Changes needed in practice. British Journal of Midwifery 1(1): 21–24.

Page L 1995 Effective group practice in midwifery: Working with women: Blackwell Science, Oxford.

Page L, Beake S, Vail A, McCourt C 2001 Clinical outcomes of one-to-one practice. British Journal of Medicine 9: 700–706.

Page L, Cooke P, Percival P 2000 Providing one-to-one care and enjoying it. In: L Page (Ed). The new midwifery: Science and sensitivity in practice. Churchill Livingstone, Edinburgh, pp. 123–140.

Pairman S 2000 Partnerships or professional friendships? In: M Kirkham (Ed). The midwife–mother relationship. Macmillan, Basingstoke.

Powell Kennedy H 2000 A model of exemplary midwifery practice: Results of a Delphi study. Journal of Midwifery and Women's Health 45(1): 4–19.

Powell Kennedy H 2004 Orchestrating normal: The art and conduct of midwifery practice. Paper presented at the Second International Conference on Normal Labour and Birth, Grange-over-Sands.

Powell Kennedy H, Rousseau A, Kane Low L 2003 An exploratory metasynthesis of midwifery practice in the United States. Midwifery 19: 2003–2214.

Powell Kennedy H, Shannon MT, Chuahorm U, Kravetz MK 2004 The landscape of caring for women: A narrative study of midwifery practice. Journal of Midwifery and Women's Health 49(1): 14–23.

Rafferty A 1995 Political leadership in nursing: The role of nursing in health-care reform. Final Report. Harkness Fellowship, May 1995.

Raimond P, Eden C 1990 Making strategy work. British Journal of Health-care Management 23(6): 11–14.

RCM 2001 Woman-centred care: A position paper. Royal College of Midwives, London.

Reed B 2002a The Albany Midwifery Practice (1). MIDIRS Midwifery Digest 12(1): 118–121.

Reed B 2002b The Albany Midwifery Practice (2). MIDIRS Midwifery Digest 12(3): 261–264.

Roberts C, Tracy S, Peat B 1999 Rates for obstetric intervention among private and public patients in Australia: Population based descriptive study. British Medical Journal 321: 137–141.

Rosener J 1990 Ways women lead. Harvard Business Review (November–December): 119–125.

Sandall J 1997 Midwives' burnout and continuity of care. British Journal of Midwifery 5(2): 106–111.

Sandall J, Davies J, Warwick C 2001 Evaluation of the Albany midwifery practice: Final report. Nightingale School of Midwifery, Kings College London.

Schindler Rising S 1998 Centering pregnancy: An interdisciplinary model of empowerment. Journal of Nurse-Midwifery 43(1): 46–54.

Simkin P 1999 Just another day in a woman's life? Women's long term perceptions of their first birth experience, Part 1. Birth 18: 203–210.

Taffinder P 1995 The new leaders: Achieving corporate transformation through dynamic leadership. Kogan Page, London.

Thiele B, Thorogood C 1997 Community Based Midwifery Program in Fremantle, WA. Centre for Research for Women, Fremantle, WA.

Thompson F 2004 Mothers and midwives: The ethical journey. Books for Midwives, Edinburgh.

Thorogood C, Thiele B, Hyde K 2002 Second Evaluation of the Community Midwifery Program. Centre for Research for Women, Freemantle, WA.

Tracy S, Tracy M 2003 Costing the cascade: Estimating the costs of increased intervention in childbirth using population data. British Journal of Obstetrics and Gynaecology 110(August): 717–724.

Tyson H (1991) Outcomes of 1001 midwife-attended home births in Toronto1983–1988. Birth 18: 14–19.

Walker K 1995 Nursing, narrativity and research: Towards a poetic and politics of orality. Contemporary Nurse 4(4): 156–163.

Warwick C 1996 Supervision and practice change at King's. In: M J Kirkham (Ed). Supervision of midwives. Books for Midwives Press, London, pp. 102–112.

Wass A 2004 Promoting health – The primary health-care approach. Harcourt Brace, Sydney.

Wiegers T, Keirse M, van der Zee J 1996 Outcome of planned home and hospital births in low risk pregnancies: Prospective study in midwifery practice in the Netherlands. British Medical Journal 131: 1309–1313.

Williams H 2003 Storied births: Narrative and organizational culture in a midwife-led birth centre. Kings College London, London.

Willis E 1983 Medical dominance: The division of labour in Australian health-care. Allen Unwin, Sydney.

Woodcock H, Read A, Moore D, Stanley F, Bower C 1990 Planned homebirths in Western Australia 1981–1987: A descriptive study. Medical Journal of Australia 153: 672–678.

World Health Organization 1986 First International Conference on Health Promotion: Ottawa Charter for Health Promotion: WHO, Geneva.

World Health Organization 1996 Care in normal birth: A practical guide. Maternal and Newborn Health/Safe Motherhood Unit, Family and Reproductive Health, WHO, Geneva.

Glossary

CAPITALISM

Capitalism is that form of economy in which the means of production (capital) are privately owned and privately controlled and labour power is purchased by the payment of money wages by the owner of capital. The goal of production is the making of profit by the sale of commodities in a competitive free market.

DISCOURSE

A discourse is patterned system of texts, messages, talk, dialogue or conversations. Discourse includes any sign and is not limited to spoken or written words. Like metanarratives discourses are neither completely true nor false. Society decides which discourses to treat as 'true' thus we say that truth is socially constructed.

DOCILE SUBJECTS

Disciplinary power induces submission by promising subjects rewards for compliance and punishments for non-compliance; this is normally done implicitly and the complying subject is then docile (Foucault 1980).

METANARRATIVE

A 'metanarrative' is a theory or story that passes itself off as a truth such as 'having a baby in a hospital under medical control is the safest way to give birth' or 'science is the best approach to solving all human problems'. Metanarratives, post-structuralists claim, are partially false and partially true, but seldom completely true.

MODERNISM AND HUMANISM

Modernism is a set of theories emerging from the Enlightenment unified under the belief that society can be perfected through the application of rational grand theories (metanarratives) coupled with science and technology. Modernist thinkers assume that there is 'truth' which can be discovered through rational investigation. In deciding the 'truth' or meaning of a text, modernists seek to know the author's meaning placing the subject at the centre of meaning-making. Humanism, which is central to modernist theory, is predicated on a belief in a dualistic subject where mind/body, reason/emotion are divided and the first term is privileged. The subject's ego is seen as an integrating controller of all parts of the self.

Humanism seeks to find one essential, universal human nature that is the basis for the claim that all humans are the same and therefore equal (Scott and Marshall 2005).

PATRIARCHY

Patriarchy is a familial-social, ideological, political system in which men, by force, direct pressure or through ritual, tradition, law, and language, customs, etiquette, education and the division of labour, determine what part women shall or shall not play, and in which the female is everywhere subsumed under the male.

POSTMODERNISM

Postmodernism is a set of sometimes conflicting theories, dating (debatably) from the 1960s. Postmodernist theories generally criticize the metanarratives of Modernism because of their inadequacies and unintended consequences (Johnson 1994). The notion that society is perfectible or that humans can know and control the world is rejected within postmodernism. Additionally, the modernist universal subject, postmodernists argue, excludes or diminishes subjects other than Western, upper class, white males (Johnson 1994). Postmodernism argues that the subject is not integrated but is fragmented and contradictory. The subject is performative in that s/he acts out various identities (Butler 1994). Postmodernism, when applied to the arts and social sciences is termed, poststructuralist.

POSTMODERNIST

A postmodernist is one who has an attitude of incredulity towards metanarratives. From a postmodernist perspective metanarratives are myths that oversimplify and blind us to subtleties, complexity and exceptions.

POWER

Power is energy which enables an individual (or a group) to be able to do or obtain what they want. Power is ethically neutral; this is consistent with Foucault's notion of power which he argued was productive; not necessarily oppressive.

POWER (DISCIPLINARY)

Professionals use a form of coercive power that Foucault named '*disciplinary power*' which operates concurrently with, and may subvert, the subject's legal power. In contrast to the way is which legal power operates openly and clearly disciplinary power seeks invisibility. Unlike legal power, disciplinary power requires the co-operation of the subject. Disciplinary power is difficult to detect, usually not becoming visible until the object of disciplinary power offers resistance (Foucault 1980).

POWER/KNOWLEDGE

Power and knowledge are self-referential and synergistic. This means that having the public accept the discipline's knowledge claims as 'true' has the effect of increasing the power of the discipline (Foucault 1980).

STRUCTURALISM

Structuralism is a theoretical approach in the arts and social sciences which is linked to modernism and post-structuralism. In general structuralism explores the relationships between fundamental elements and some higher 'structures' which are built upon them. In sociology the reference is to the individuals in relation to each other as the foundations of some larger social institution. In linguistics the fundamental elements are words or signs which carry the meaning of language between people. Saussure argued that a language can be described in terms of a basic set of rules which govern the combination of sounds to produce meanings. The word 'meaning' here is very close to the word 'truth'. For Lévi-Strauss the fundamental structures are concepts or ideas. Concepts are language-based and encoded in the mind. For Lévi-Strauss these internal concepts can always be understood as binary oppositions (for example man/woman; reason/emotion) (Scott and Marshall 2005).

STRUCTURALISM (POST-)

Post-structuralism has been considered in two main ways: one concerns the subject and power, for example, in the work of Michel Foucault. The other main way is post structuralism as exemplified in the work of Jacques Derrida, which is a direct criticism of structuralism. Linguistic post-structuralists have shown that the meanings (truths) cannot be fixed. This is because the supposedly foundational terms upon which the meanings depend are equally contingent and unstable (Calhoun 2002). In the view of post-structuralists 'truth' is, therefore, contingent so that what comes to be accepted as 'truth' is a product of relations of power (Foucault 1980).

SURVEILLANCE AND THE GAZE

Surveillance, meaning observation, depends upon what Foucault called *'the gaze'*. This gaze of medical surveillance is a pre-requisite for medical power. The subjects of medical power must make their bodies open to the medical gaze. Patients give up their bodily secrets in the belief that medical power can control disease (Foucault 1980).

References

Calhoun CJ 2002 Contemporary Sociological Theory. Oxford, Blackwell.

Foucault M 1980 Power/knowledge: selected interviews. Pantheon, New York.

Johnson P 1994 Feminism as radical humanism. Sydney, Allen and Unwin.

Scott J and Marshall G 2005 A Dictionary of Sociology. Oxford University Press, Oxford.

Index

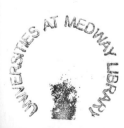